WHY LOVE HEALS

HEALS

Mind-Body-Spirit
Medicine

Also by Dean Shrock, Ph.D.

DOCTOR'S ORDERS: GO FISHING

Heartfelt Intent Publications
Eagle Point, Oregon 97524

Front book cover photograph by Philip Wolfmueller

Back cover photograph by Shelly Shrock

Book cover graphics and layout design by Roger Vilsack, Vilsack Productions, Arlington VA.

ISBN 978-0-9819751-0-8

For my wife

Shelly Shrock

Who I love more each day.
I don't know what I've done
to deserve her and her pure
heart. She is, indeed, my
soulmate, and makes my life
so worthwhile.

We Are Water and Spirit

You can look into a mirror and see your image
Water reflects your image too
But unlike a mirror you must get close to the water and
yourself to see the reflection
And you and the water must be still and untroubled by
outside forces
And just as water may exist as a liquid, solid or vapor
You can undergo continual transformation too
Depending on your state of consciousness
You can choose to close your heart
And become hard and cold as ice
Or become sparkling diamonds on the branches of the tree
of life
Or protect and guard the life which exists beneath the surface
For it is only when we are willing to go beneath the surface
Into the stillness and depth of our being that we truly find
ourselves
And create the authentic path our stream should follow
As a stream of water flows over and around stones making
beautiful sounds
Your blood stream can flow over obstacles, become as
destructive as a tsunami
Or choose to vaporize and rise above life's difficulties
Ready to fall back, when needed,
As gentle rain softening the soil of life
One day every blood stream will find its way to the endless
sea of life
Where you will be reborn as white crystals
Which descend slowly and gently onto the frozen ground
When the world experiences a drought of love
Forming a blank canvas upon which the world can now create a
work of art

Acknowledgments

This book is dedicated to my wife, Shelly. But I also must acknowledge her support in the writing of this book. She has typed and retyped every page, and I truly appreciate her insights and suggestions.

I, of course, am eternally grateful for my spiritual guide, Ken McCaulley. Ken was my best friend and mentor until he died in 1999. He has continued to give me great support and guidance in writing *Why Love Heals*.

I also need to acknowledge John the Baptist, who I was able to speak with through the channeling of the medium, Sharon Bauer. I couldn't appreciate these conversations more, and his understanding of why love heals.

I want to thank Sharon Bauer with all of my heart. She has allowed me to talk weekly with Ken McCaulley, John the Baptist, and her spirit guide, David. I value her support and friendship greatly.

I wish to acknowledge my good friend, Dr. Jodine Turner, who has offered valuable assistance in the editing of this book. She is an author, and trained with Dr. James Lynch, whose research led me to investigate and write *Why Love Heals*.

Lastly, I want to thank James Barrett, Bernie Siegel, and Len Laskow for their thoughtful feedback of an earlier manuscript of *Why Love Heals*. And I want to thank my friends, Ralph Napolitano and Krystalya Marie' for their dedicated support, patience, and marketing expertise. I love you all.

Table of Contents

Introduction

My purpose for writing this book was to look more closely at a conclusion I had made in my last book, *Doctor's Orders: Go Fishing*. As Director of Mind-Body Medicine for a large group of cancer centers, I was very interested in the "will to live", and how it could impact patients' quality of life, and, potentially, the length of their life. I am certain, for reasons I will yet explain, that teaching and encouraging this will to live as part of their medical treatment, was effective. However, our research concluded that they lived longer because they felt listened to and supported. In short, they felt loved and cared for.

This was also Dr. Dean Ornish's conclusion with heart disease. I cannot speak highly enough about Ornish's research and the books he has written as a result of his groundbreaking work. His research has been published in the world's leading medical journals, including *The Lancet* and *The Journal of the American Medical Association*. He and his colleagues found that you could stop, or begin to reverse heart disease, following lifestyle changes in nutrition, exercise, and stress management. Even severe coronary heart disease often begins to reverse when making these lifestyle changes, without drugs or surgery!

Very interestingly, after twenty years of research and practice as a cardiologist, Ornish wrote in his book, *Love and Survival*, that no other factor in medicine, "*not diet, not smoking, not exercise, not stress, not genetics, not drugs, not surgery*", affects our health, quality and length of life more than feeling loved and cared for. He believes that opening your heart means opening your heart anatomically, emotionally, and spiritually. This means that medical knowledge must be integrated with a deeper, ancient wisdom: that peace and well-being come from within. We need to open our heart to this truth of who we are. He states that heart disease needs to be treated with altruism, compassion, and love, "not just unclogging arteries."

Ornish's conclusions were given strong support by the research of Dr. James Lynch, a psychologist on faculty at the University of Maryland. His thirty years of research with patients having high blood pressure and heart disease concluded that heartfelt listening and communication were vital for heart health. When people felt heard and understood, their bodies responded in a far healthier way than when they were unable to speak from their heart. This is documented well in his many books, including, *A Cry Unheard: New Insights into the Medical Consequences of Loneliness*. Both Lynch and Ornish demonstrated clearly that loneliness and isolation contribute to all forms of premature death.

So, based on this research, we could conclude that people are healthier and live longer when they feel heard, understood, loved, and cared for. This shouldn't be so surprising for a number of reasons. There would appear to be good common sense in the ability of love to heal. Nurses, in particular, have been identified as dispensing TLC (tender loving care) as part of their healing practice. How about the role of the doctor's bedside manner? Every spiritual system espouses the role of love as the way to improve all aspects of life. Who doesn't know that positive feelings such as joy and forgiveness, and a positive attitude promote health and healing?

In this book I explore some of the reasons why we don't take psycho-social-spiritual factors into greater account. This was not the case for all of recorded history prior to the seventeenth century. But then Sir Isaac Newton and physics took a decidedly mechanical view of the universe. And since that time, thought, reason, and science have dominated what we determine as fact or truth.

We could certainly say that this isn't such a bad idea. Who wants their healthcare provider basing a medical decision on dreams, visions, or spiritual insight vs. controlled laboratory research? However, this strict reliance on current approaches to research and healthcare is questionable for a number of reasons. One, we're doing relatively little psycho-social-spiritual research as it relates to health. Two, healthcare is dominated by the pharmaceutical industry. Three, quantum physics research demonstrates that consciousness (including, but going much farther than, the placebo effect) has a far greater impact on reality than previously understood. Truth is a lot more subjective than we really understand or want to admit. Unless a study is truly "double-blind", which is seldom the case, there is real reason to question the results. Four, medical training has not adequately addressed these much broader psycho-social-spiritual factors. Truly effective healthcare must include these variables, and I will discuss this throughout the chapters of *Why Love Heals*.

There is a huge database from university Prevention Research Centers and schools of Preventive Medicine and Public Health demonstrating the health benefits of an improved lifestyle, especially with exercise and nutrition. We know that two thirds of deaths from all illness under age 65 are preventable. More than one half of all hospital admissions can be prevented by changes in lifestyle. Why are we ignoring this? The reason is that we have come to look to the medical profession as having all the answers, even though medical students are not required to study even the basic components of wellness: exercise, nutrition, and stress management. It is a very recent phenomenon that many medical schools now have course work in these subjects, as well as spirituality and health. But they are almost always offered as electives, which means that medical students are not required to study these subjects as part of their medical degree.

In this book I make what I believe is a very strong case for why love heals. But I know that most people will only do what their doctors tell them. And their doctors are not even telling them about the importance of exercise and nutrition, let alone about psychological and spiritual factors! I must add that a notable recent exception is in the practice of integrative and functional medicine. These medical approaches provide more comprehensive assessment, treatment, prevention, and management of disease than conventional medical care, especially with chronic disease.

In the *Textbook of Functional Medicine*, Dr. David Jones and Sheila Quinn state in their chapter, "Why Functional Medicine":

> Despite the fact that non-genetic factors that are *modifiable* – including diet, overweight, inactivity, and environmental exposures such as smoking – account for 70-90% of mortality in the U.S., physician education, training, and reimbursement are

most often focused on treating disease using drugs and surgery rather than comprehensive patient-centered treatments focused on the individual. For example, as reported in a study published in the *British Medical Journal*, clinical questions in primary care can be categorized into a limited number of generic types and frequency. The four most common question types were:

1. What is the drug of choice for condition x?
2. What is the cause of symptom x?
3. What test is indicated in situation x?
4. What is the dose of drug x?

This shortsighted approach to health care should give us all cause for serious concern, because it is perpetuating a system that is far too costly and increasingly ineffective for the prevention and management of chronic diseases whose root causes are to be found in a much more complex perspective on patients' lives.

Jones and Quinn state that these lifestyle root causes, including stress and social isolation, are "the greatest threats to American health".

Dr. Andrew Weil states in the first sentence of his preface to *Integrative Oncology*, which he edited with Dr. Donald Abrams, that Integrative Medicine "takes account of the whole person (body, mind, spirit), as well as all aspects of lifestyle." Integrative medicine includes practitioners in conventional medical care with proven, effective complementary approaches, such as acupuncture, yoga, exercise, nutrition, psychotherapy, meditation, and massage. Dr. Weil believes that we need to shift the focus of health care from disease management to "the innate healing potentials of the human organism."

I was very pleased to view the testimony on February 26, 2009 of the hearings for the United States Committee on Health, Labor, and Pensions. Here, physicians Dr. Mark Hyman (who is on the faculty of the Institute for Functional Medicine and is Editor in Chief of *Alternative Therapies in Health and Medicine*, where my research was published), Dr. Mehmet Oz, Dr. Dean Ornish, and Dr. Andrew Weil led a panel titled, "Integrative Care: A Pathway to a Healthier Nation." They clearly and eloquently stressed the need for preventative approaches to health, and the promotion of wellness. It was extremely heartening to have seen the very favorable support from Senators Harkin and Mikulski, who chaired this government hearing.

At some point we simply have to look at the dismal success of treating chronic disease. Almost everyone has a chronic disease from which they suffer, and which will eventually take their life. Chronic diseases are by far the leading causes of death in the world, representing 60% of all deaths. Clearly current healthcare practices need to change. In fact, medical errors are the third leading cause of death in the United States behind heart disease and cancer. Something must be done to improve this. The remedy is lifestyle. This is no longer a radical consideration. Far too much research and common sense exist to deny the benefit of nutrition, exercise, environmental factors, and stress management. And, so, this book has become an opportunity for me to speak my truth.

Speak Your Truth

In 1993 I attended a weekend workshop by Dr. Joan Borysenko. She had been an inspiration for me for several years. I had contacted her initially related to my doctoral dissertation. In fact she sent me an audiocassette of a meditation she used as Director of the Mind/Body Clinic she co-founded with Dr. Herbert Benson at Beth Israel/Deaconess Medical Center in Boston, which I used in my research.

Her best-selling 1987 book, *Minding the Body, Mending the Mind*, was an appealing blend of science and common sense. It was just what I was looking for to help me in developing my program teaching cancer patients and their families how to cope with the diagnosis and treatment of cancer. Her 1990 book, *Guilt is the Teacher, Love is the Lesson*, became one of my all time favorites. It was more than a blend of science and common sense; I can say now that it touched my soul.

I didn't fully understand this at the time, but now I value her wisdom and courage more than ever. She was a licensed clinical psychologist, with graduate study in psychopharmacology, worked as a cancer cell biologist for ten years, had post-doctoral degrees in cancer cell biology, behavioral medicine, and psychoneuro-immunology. Yet here she was in this workshop talking about spirituality, which, of course, she wrote about extensively in her books. I remember asking her how she was able to do this. How, as a scientist, was she so comfortable talking about spiritual issues? She signed her book, "With best wishes – Speak your truth!" I've always remembered this.

I learned in graduate school that whatever I said or wrote had to be supported with primary research. Anecdotal evidence or personal opinion was akin to heresy. This was also the case, of course, when I was working in medical centers or with medical doctors for most of my career. But a crazy thing happened along the way: I discovered intuition and that there truly is a spiritual side to life. It was indeed a blessing, but how do you function as a scientifically trained healthcare professional and speak this truth?

In reviewing piles and piles of articles and notes I've taken over the years, in preparation for this book, I was pleasantly reminded that there have been many others who have spoken their truth eloquently. Dr. Larry Dossey has been incredible this way. He has been a tremendous resource for me, and I'm sure for many others. His earliest books: *Space, Time and Medicine; Beyond Illness; Recovering the Soul; Meaning and Medicine*; and *Healing Words* were (like Joan Borysenko) this unique blend of scientific data, common sense, and spiritual insight. Of course, all of his books have had this quality, but these were what I read early on as I was developing psychological services for cancer centers. His books became instrumental in introducing the role of religious practice and prayer in medical schools. Today nearly 80 medical schools have such classes, with Dossey's books among their textbooks.

Notable others who were comfortable discussing spiritual practices as part of healing included Dr. Rachel Naomi Remen. In a presentation titled, "Care for the

Soul", she taught very clearly that we are not just our bodies, and that our sense of meaning is our greatest protection against the challenges of life. The separation of the sacred from the secular (even more than the separation of mind and body) is the great wound that needs to be healed. Part of the wound and flaw of our current system is that we're not caring for the soul. She noted that shamans refer to illness as "soul loss." Whenever you stop "singing" (lose meaning, connection, purpose, and zest for life), soul loss and illness result.

My study of quantum physics gave me additional insights into spirituality and health. I am especially indebted to Lynn McTaggart and her books, *The Field* and *The Intention Experiment* for her unique ability to clarify the science of quantum physics. Her website is filled with health and related information (www.theintentionexperiment.com). I also must credit Ken Wilber and his 1982 book, *The Holographic Paradigm and Other Paradoxes.* This is where I first heard of physicist, Dr. David Bohm, and his belief that there is an infinite sea of energy that underlies all of physical reality. He proposed that everything is a form of energy. Physical matter is a very gross form, but there are other forms that are more subtle that interrelate with all other forms of energy and matter. Underlying all of these energy fields is a Primary Reality, which is a source of all other realities.

Bohm claimed that our physical perception of material reality has conditioned us to think of ourselves as being separate from other human beings and other forms of matter. But, the fact is, we are all interconnected. And because of the interconnection of all realities, any one form is potentially all-knowledgeable. However, one's physical senses set limits on what can be perceived. We perceive as real that which we have been conditioned to believe is true.

Bohm suggested that any ideas and thoughts that do not support these conditioned beliefs create a "pressure", and that "you accept as true any statement that will relieve that pressure." Therefore, to have a clearer picture of reality, the first priority is to change our beliefs. He notes that our beliefs about our separateness is really a result of such pressures. These include fear, gain, greed, compromise, trade-offs, and pressures to achieve. This "corruption" of our consciousness could be healed by people having a "oneness" understanding, and working together to change this collective consciousness to one of responsibility toward humankind.

Bohm, in collaboration with the Indian sage Krishnamurti, believed that meditation is a means to transform the mind of conditioned thoughts. By quieting oneself through passive, focused attention, consciousness can be transformed. In a deeply relaxed, meditative state, the brain becomes quiet and sympathetic with the underlying universal frequency pattern. This allows a new means to perceive reality, an alternative way of knowing, which can reprogram the brain.

Thinking is a filtering process and distorts true reality. Enlightenment, according to Bohm and Krishnamurti, is the channeling of the universal force to operate through us. They extend this proposition, blending physics, religion and mysticism. This "wholeness" which links the entire universe is a force of compassion, an active concern for all of creation. They conclude, "In short, the energy itself is love... the ultimate nature of the universe is an energy of love."

Quantum physics and its concepts of "entanglement" and "nonlocality" were excellent support for my definition of love as oneness and why love heals. It added science to a consideration of love. Love was not just an emotion or something that belonged to the metaphysical or philosophical. Love is a universal, all-pervasive energy that flows through everything. When your thoughts and behaviors resonate in harmony with this Primary Reality of harmony and order, health is a natural consequence. When we experience any sense of separateness, we restrict the flow of this life-giving energy, and disharmony and disease result.

There is strong reason and evidence to believe that thoughts and feelings such as separation vs. oneness; of fear vs. love; of despair vs. hope, constrict the flow of a Life Force or quantum energy, which lead to illness. These negative thoughts and feelings are another way to define stress. This is why all illness is stress-related in some way.

I want to conclude this introduction to *Why Love Heals* by stating that research and science are methods to determine truth, but meditation and intuition are a way to understand a deeper truth. I'll reveal throughout the book some of my personal experiences, including now being able to communicate with my deceased friend, Ken McCaulley, once again.

I have learned that the truth lies within everyone. I have been blessed to have had Ken's psychic ability to teach me this early on. And now, through the psychic ability of a new dear friend, Sharon Bauer, I have Ken and other spiritual teachers to assist me. At some point during our many meetings, Sharon went into a trance state, and began to channel the Ascended Master, John the Baptist.

Chapter 10 includes some of the conversations John and I have had over the past couple of months. John explained himself as a collective spiritual consciousness, the same as Abraham is for Esther and Jerry Hicks. These spiritual beings are committed to teaching us to love ourselves, and that we are greatly valued "on the other side of the veil".

I asked John why love heals. Here was his immediate response: "It's because of the vibration of love. It's the energy that is attached to love that heals. Love is the vibration of the soul. It's a direct connection from us on the other side to their soul... Once you've healed and touched the soul, then the body will follow." In summary, he pleaded with us to raise the universal consciousness by connecting with Divine Source; and when we do, health is a byproduct.

I then asked John to say whatever he would like to say to conclude the book. His final statements were: "Humans are always, and will always be connected to Divine Source, the source of love of God. Humans will always be love. Humans must experience emotion (both positive and negative) on this side of the veil in order to grow... If they could just only do this one simple task – to truly learn to love and forgive the negative – and if they could truly love that, and go through a daily ritual, awareness, or task that brings them back into remembrance of who they are, Dean, this is the greatest message I would want to give."

This is my truth that I want to share with you now.

Chapter 1 - How It All Began

My father died my first day at college. The Dean of Students came into my dorm room with the phone message from my mother. Arrangements had already been made for a friend of the family to pick me up and drive me to the airport for a flight home that night.

My father had been scheduled for a routine operation to repair a heart valve the day after I left for school. We were told that the surgery was successful, but something happened in the recovery room, and my father never regained consciousness.

When I left home, there was no thought other than I would see him in a month or so when I returned for Mother's Day. Now I was surrounded by friends and family, not really grasping that my father was no longer here. I remember how touched I was by the support of my many high school friends, in particular.

My real concern was for my mother. My twin brother was away at college also. Thank goodness, my sister, who was a senior in high school, was there to be with my Mom. There were so many things to think about and attend to. But I had to return to college the next weekend and begin my classes one week late. My mother was clear that this had to be my focus.

I had always been a good student. I guess I had always been a good kid. All of us were. My dad saw to that. Upon reflection, I think of him mostly as a disciplinarian. I remember him telling me that he never cared if we ever thought of him as a friend; we were going to learn discipline. I learned early on that whatever he said, you accepted without question.

You never said "No" to my father. I tried that once, and got slapped around pretty good. He definitely didn't believe in sparing the rod. Even my mother could come after us with her shoe or the washing stick. But dad clearly ruled the roost. And now he wasn't there to tell me what to do. I didn't realize that I would spend the rest of my life trying to earn his love. This would be instrumental in my quest to learn why love heals.

I had attended an excellent public high school in Pittsburgh, Pennsylvania where most of the students went on to college. I had a "high honor" grade-point average, and received a scholarship to attend Fenn College of Engineering in Cleveland, Ohio. However, as good a student as I was, I wasn't really prepared for the rigor of my college studies.

Maybe taking 20 credits a quarter was too much. Or maybe being on my own affected my study habits. Anyhow, my grades soon suffered, and I lost my scholarship after the first year.

Actually, I'm pretty sure that after eighteen years of being under my father's thumb, it was time to express my independence. I was now out drinking beer with my new friends most nights of the week, eventually got thrown out of the dorm for being a "flagrant disobeyer of authority", and joined a fraternity, which contributed that much more to my attempt to break free of my father's influence. Of course, it was only demonstrating that he still controlled my life. However, this sense of independence allowed me the freedom to explore many new opportunities, culminating in my interest in mind-body-spirit medicine.

I changed my field of study from engineering to education and finally to psychology, before graduating with a C average. I had had a great time socially, but now I was on my own again, penniless, and had to get a job with only an undergraduate degree in psychology.

Even though I had this low grade-point average, I was remarkably self-confident. I pretty much had been able to accomplish whatever I had wanted in most of my life. I knew you just had to work at it. And now I rather calmly asked myself, "What would you like to do?" At the time I wasn't particularly concerned about my knowledge or training in choosing a job. I had come to terms with the fact that I had to support myself, and as long as I was going to get up every morning to go to work, I should find something I'd enjoy doing.

I had no background in the stock market, but I thought being a stockbroker would be interesting. I also had an interest in clothing. I had worked as a salesperson in a men's clothing store while in high school and even opened my own little store in the fraternity house, where I sold a few shirts supplied from that store in Pittsburgh. I settled on becoming a buyer for a major private department store in downtown Cleveland, only twelve blocks from Fenn College, which by then had become Cleveland State University.

I started out in their training program earning five hundred dollars a month working in men's furnishings and sportswear. Although that salary seems very meager now, in 1968 it was enough to manage my limited needs, and I shared an apartment with fraternity brothers near the fraternity house. I had a pretty nice life at age 24.

After a year and a half of training with the department store I left and opened a little clothing store near the university. I acquired a Small Business Administration loan for twenty five thousand dollars, and opened my small store across the street from Cleveland State selling mostly blue jeans and T-shirts and related items, including "pipes" and "papers".

My life changed dramatically. I had always been conservative in my dress. I wore a suit and tie to work every day. In high school we commonly shopped at Brooks Brothers, and our basic wardrobe was their blue shirt and khaki colored slacks. But now I was selling and wearing bell-bottom jeans, tie-dyed T-shirts, a leather jacket with fringe hanging from the sleeves, and moccasins. I grew a fu-man-chu mustache, quit getting haircuts, and started smoking "dope". Yes, I inhaled.

My circle of friends also began to change, and I was meeting lots of interesting people in the store. We were open seven days a week, noon to midnight, and were right next door to a college bar and record store. I quickly learned to like my new lifestyle.

But thank God I had the training at the department store. People tended to think that it was glamorous to own a store, or as they often referred to it, a boutique. But it was a lot of work. We had a shoestring budget, to say the least. I had to do everything to stay afloat. Eventually I hired as many as three people to help me, but my life revolved around that store for the first year.

Then I bought a second store in Cleveland Heights on Coventry Road. This was the place to be in Cleveland if you were young or young-minded. Although it might sound at first that I was now going to be even busier, I was successful enough to be able to hire very capable people to help me run the stores, and I shortened our work days and hours.

Just as I had cut loose in college following my dad's death, I continued my free lifestyle in the 70's. Make no mistake; I worked very hard in running the stores. But I also played hard and had great fun. I sold concert tickets for Belkin Productions out of the stores, and attended a rock concert just about every weekend. I met numbers of entertainers who were in town to perform. I even became friends with Mark Farner from the band, Grand Funk Railroad.

By 1974 the economy was getting worse and worse, and business dropped considerably. Actually, I had already closed the first store by then due to three armed robberies. While I had this great social life, the business was becoming very stressful. Maybe it was a stroke of luck that there was a major fire two doors away which smoke-damaged everything in my store in 1977. I decided to take the insurance settlement, pay my debts, and start yet another new life.

If losing my dad, going off to college, learning to live on my own, owning the clothing stores, and changing my lifestyle dramatically wasn't enough, 1977 was to become the absolute turning point in my life. In the summer of 1977 I met a man named Ken McCaulley, who taught a self-improvement program that he called HELP, which stood for Human Expansion Through Liberated Potential. But, first I need to back up and explain another major change in my life, which led to meeting Ken and why this changed my life so completely. Ken was to become my best teacher in coming to understand the need to love.

My Interest In Parapsychology

I had become good friends with one of my fraternity brothers, Terry, and his wife, Mary. Mary was probably as good a female friend as I had at that time. And "out of the blue" one day she told me that she saw ghosts. If she was not such a good friend, I probably would have written this off as craziness, which is largely what her husband did. While I didn't have any experience with this, I wanted to be supportive, and at least listen to what she had to say. I knew she wasn't lying or making this up. She had no reason to do that. So, I accepted that maybe she really did see ghosts, but who knows.

As we continued to talk about her experience and interest in this psychic stuff, she told me that she read tarot cards, which also was new to me. I was surprised that while I was attempting to be supportive of her, I found myself becoming more curious and interested. I was especially fascinated in learning that she could use the tarot cards and her own psychic ability to foretell the future.

I have to admit that I was embarrassed at first by my interest in all of this stuff. What would my "normal" friends think? I still had contact with my college friends, and they had never talked about any of this. Or, like Terry, they thought this was "kooky" or worse.

As my curiosity grew, I found myself reading books on the subject. I especially remember my interest in the Jane Roberts' books, *Seth Speaks* and *The Nature of Personal Reality*. These books said that you literally create your own reality. This was all very strange and new to me, but I found this information and my friendship with Mary growing deeper and deeper.

Then I began to meet more people who shared this interest, which led to my attending workshops and related presentations that were decidedly metaphysical. This surprised me, too, because I didn't really have any particular religious or spiritual beliefs. Who would believe that I now was thinking and talking about ghosts, tarot cards, psychics, reincarnation, and spirit guides. And then I met Ken McCaulley.

Ken McCaulley

Ken's HELP program was six two-hour evening classes that looked at learned beliefs about who we are, and what limits our ability to be truly happy and healthy. Each lecture ended with a guided imagery exercise, where you closed your eyes and imagined yourself relaxed and now able to function under your own control, free of these learned limitations. I remember feeling so good when class ended at nine o'clock that I wasn't going to just go home and go to bed. I had to go out and enjoy how good I really felt. The information was very stimulating, and the "mental exercises" were better than dope.

I had lots of questions, and Ken always was willing to take time for me. I still owned the clothing store at the time, but I would arrange to leave and meet with Ken to talk at length about all kinds of things.

It turned out that Ken had been psychic all of his life. Unfortunately, his family didn't understand his ability, and actually thought he was mentally disturbed. His father called him "the crazy bastard." Eventually Ken went to a psychiatrist for treatment. He was blessed that this doctor had some knowledge in the area of parapsychology, and recommended that Ken read numbers of books to help him understand and accept his "extra sensory perception."

Ken had a fascinating background, which I learned over the next few months. He was a voracious reader. He told me that he would read one or two books daily. I don't remember the exact order of things, but he had a master's degree in education, taught in a public school, was an ordained Presbyterian minister, and had a tremendous interest in parapsychology, which he also taught in adult education classes. I quickly learned that Ken's greatest gift and drive was as a genuine seeker of truth. Ken and I soon became best friends and business partners, and worked together teaching his program for the next ten years.

Ken was the first to introduce me to guided imagery, where (like self-hypnosis) you imagine a desired outcome in order to improve any area of your life. Because of my training and experience with Ken and guided imagery I returned to college in 1980, and earned my Ph.D. in psychology from the University of Akron in 1986. My doctoral dissertation was titled, *Relaxation, Guided Imagery, and Wellness*.

Carl Simonton

Then in 1987 I met Dr. Carl Simonton when I interned at his weeklong cancer program in Pacific Palisades, California. I was especially interested in working with Carl because of his strong interest in guided imagery. He had cancer patients imagine their immune systems working properly: visualizing white blood cells easily removing cancer cells from the body. Ken and Carl were two of the wisest men I have ever met. They taught me much more about health and life, and are directly responsible for my current interest in why love heals.

The greatest tool that both Ken and Carl taught was to develop your intuition. As I said, Ken had been psychic all of his life, and spent considerable time studying and attempting to understand his and others' ability to "know" something without any objective evidence. He taught meditation and intuition as part of his HELP course.

Before long, Ken and I began to meditate and practice our intuition daily. At some point Ken began to go into a trance-like state and speak a truth and wisdom that was far beyond his current knowledge and intellect. For approximately seven years, I spoke with this "wisdom" daily, and I value this experience more than I could possibly explain. Ken's course had a class called "Manifesting Love", where he asked people to consider their life purpose and related questions like: Who am I? Where did I come from? Why am I here? And it all seemed to revolve around love. This was certainly the consistent message of Ken's inner wisdom.

Now I knew that there was another way to gain knowledge and insight: I could focus my attention inward and get information about any question I had. It was very much like the religious and philosophical admonition to "go within". We have access to all information within ourselves.

Similarly, Carl taught how the unconscious mind communicates with the conscious self through feelings, dreams, and intuition. He encouraged people to practice mental relaxation, and then open themselves to receive information about their feelings, motivations, and behavior that would help them in their healing process. Carl believed that healing depended on one's attitudes, beliefs, and choices. And insight and information about this could come from the unconscious "inner guide" or "inner advisor". I'll say much more about this later.

One of the things that started Carl on his path to take a more psychological approach to cancer care was an observation he made as a radiation oncologist about his patients. Medical care essentially is based on a medical diagnosis. Once physicians know your diagnosis, they know what to do to treat you. However, people with the same diagnosis, getting the same treatment, in fact, can have very different outcomes, which is what Carl observed with his patients. Those who had a stronger "will to live" appeared to be exerting some influence over the course of their disease, and were doing better and living longer than patients who showed a greater apathy, depression, and attitude of giving up. This led Carl and his wife Stephanie, who had a background in psychology and motivational counseling, to develop a "whole-person" approach to cancer:

> It is our central premise that an illness is not purely a physical problem but rather a problem of the whole person, that it includes not only body but also mind and emotions. We believe that emotional and mental states play a significant role both in *susceptibility* to disease, including cancer, and in *recovery* from all disease. We believe that cancer is often an indication of problems elsewhere in an individual's life, problems aggravated or compounded by a series of stresses six to eighteen months prior to the onset of cancer. The cancer

patient has typically responded to these
problems and stresses with a deep sense of
hopelessness, or "giving up". This
emotional response, we believe, in turn
triggers a set of physiological responses that
suppress the body's natural defenses and
make it susceptible to producing abnormal
cells.

This citation from Stephanie and Carl's book,
Getting Well Again, was music to my ears. I had read the
book prior to working with Carl, and meeting him and
seeing how he implemented this mind-body-spirit
approach to cancer care was very meaningful and
inspiring. It was in this first week of meeting one another
that Carl and I planned on a lifetime of collaboration.

I was employed at this time as a staff psychologist
at a rehab hospital just outside of State College,
Pennsylvania. When I returned from my internship at the
Simonton Cancer Center, my hospital asked me to write a
protocol for a cancer program where I could use the
Simonton approach as part of this protocol. As a result I
returned for another internship that year to help prepare
for teaching and researching the Simonton method.

As it turned out, the rehab hospital didn't follow
through with the program. But the radiation oncologists in
State College who were going to refer their cancer
patients to the proposed program asked me to develop one
for them and their physician management group of cancer
centers, which at that time were primarily in
Pennsylvania. And this began an eleven-year experience
of developing, teaching, and researching a wellness-based
program for cancer patients and their families, with a
decided emphasis on the will to live.

Chapter 2 - The Will To Live

A "will to live" means that people have a desire and reason to live. Something to look forward to. Something that grabs and focuses their attention on wanting to live in order, for example, to see their children get married, to see their grandchildren born, or to complete some special project. And the reason they wanted to live didn't have to be positive. I'm certain that a number of patients I've worked with lived longer than their medical prognoses because they wanted to live to make someone else's life miserable. To be sure, I'll explain at length later in this book why a positive reason to live is healthier than a negative one, but for now, please appreciate that your will to live and your attitude can affect your physical health.

While this may seem like simple common sense, I joke that science doesn't use common sense. Science necessitates that for something to be true it must be objectively measurable through rigidly controlled experiments or research. Ethically and legally, physicians and other professionally trained healthcare providers can only tell you to do something if there is significant scientific research supporting their treatment approach. Prior to the Simontons' research, which was published in 1981 in the *Medical Journal of Australia*, very little other research had been done in the world looking at psychological factors with cancer.

A notable exception was Dr. Larry LeShan, a psychologist, who researched and reported in a number of studies that cancer patients had far greater feelings of hopelessness than patients without cancer. His strong message to counter these feelings and to affect the course of their disease was to find this will to live, or as he defined it, to find their own unique song to sing. LeShan and the Simontons believed that the goal was not to extend life, but to enrich it. However, their work and research were not well received within the medical community. It was not strong enough statistically or in methodology to be a legitimate consideration in cancer patient treatment and care.

Not only was there not enough sound research, but at that time, the idea that any psychological factor could affect any physical process was simply unacceptable, if not impossible. Prior to new research in the 1970's in a field of study called psychoneuroimmunology, it had always been believed that the immune system functioned independently of any other bodily system. This meant that the immune system could not be affected by the brain or any process associated with the central nervous system. Thus, if the brain is not connected to the immune system (the system most identified with fighting disease), how could any psychological factor affect the onset or course of disease? It couldn't. And to this day, medical science and physicians still wrestle with, and largely reject, the fact that psychological factors, including the will to live, are fundamental to one's health.

So, working in medical settings where I had to support what I taught with scientific research became a major challenge for me. I knew that I couldn't deny the impact of psychosocial factors. And I knew, because of my work and experience with Ken McCaulley, that there was so much more to life and health than could possibly be explained by current research. But I reconciled myself to be very grateful to have the opportunity to help these cancer patients and their families as best I could. What I learned from this experience caught me by surprise.

One of the first things I learned was that if I sounded too scientific, people couldn't relate to what I wanted to teach them, which was primarily at first about the will to live and guided imagery. What I did find helpful was to tell stories and draw on common life experiences to help explain the role of the will to live and how it potentially could impact their quality and length of life. I explained that there wasn't much research to support these subjects, but there also wasn't research to prove that they didn't work. There simply was very little research.

Actually, the probability was, and sadly still is, that physicians have little or no formal training in psychology and wellness. The research today actually is overwhelming that these lifestyle approaches are critical for our health. Consider that the American Cancer Society claims that one-third of all cancer deaths are caused by poor diet and physical activity. One-third more are related to tobacco. And they don't even give a percent for stress-related causes! Only ten percent are genetic. Two thirds of deaths from all illness under age 65 are preventable. More than one half of all hospital admissions can be prevented by changes in lifestyle. Clearly you can see that we need a healthcare system that recognizes the need for trained healthcare professionals to educate and provide these non-drug health approaches.

But back to my point about my dilemma in teaching cancer patients and families about these wellness approaches in cancer centers where there was little understanding or regard for the viability and seriousness of treatments other than radiation, chemotherapy, and surgery. It is well understood that one's thoughts and feelings can change blood pressure, heart rate, and how we can worry ourselves sick. Feeling happy or sad, relaxed or tense, or any change in feelings literally affects how we function physically. Who has never heard about the power of positive thinking? Who doesn't know that laughter is good medicine? Or that without hope, people perish? And even though there wasn't much research about the will to live, who doesn't know that a strong will to live makes a difference in your health? People knew from their own experience, that stress, nutrition, and exercise directly affected their health. So, even if there was limited research, or their doctors hadn't told them to do it, there was sound reason to complement their medical treatments with these non-medical approaches.

I found that people really responded to the adage, "When you're busy doing something you like to do that you tend to forget your aches and pains." I told my patients stories like the one about my friend Bob, who often couldn't walk very far before he'd have to sit down and rest. He lived on a large acreage, and would have to get around on his ATV. But when a special mushroom was growing on his property, he could walk for hours searching for these mushrooms and digging them up – without any of the heart and respiratory problems he normally would have.

The story I almost always told was about deer hunting. I was born in central Pennsylvania. I grew up knowing that there was very little in life that had more meaning to my father, uncles, and cousins than deer hunting. I am not exaggerating. In fact to this day, public schools in most of Pennsylvania are closed the first day of buck and doe season!

So, I would ask our patients, "Even if you were really sick, so sick that you couldn't even get out of bed, but it was the first day of buck season, where would most of you be?" Almost in unison they would reply, "In the woods". There was no way you were going to keep a true deer hunter out of the woods in deer season. And no matter how sick they felt, they were going to feel better for having gone hunting. And the fact is that up to two-thirds of our patients receiving radiation missed their treatments during the first week of buck season!

I have to admit that this caught me quite off guard, but I loved it. It made my teaching them about the importance of a will to live much easier than if I cited books full of research. Believe me, I knew about the problem using anecdotal evidence in the medical community to support my position, and, in this case, with something as serious as cancer. But I got my patients' attention with it, and it served to build a rapport that I also was to learn could have its own healing effects.

Have Fun 1x Daily

I explained to patients that we (speaking for myself and the cancer centers) were quite serious about wanting them to incorporate fun into their daily lives as part of the treatment for their cancer, and also as part of a way to help families cope. At some point we actually handed out calendars at Christmas time that had a facsimile of a doctor's prescription. It read, "Doctor's Orders: Have fun 1X daily". It had 365 refills. And it was signed by their radiation oncologist. While I used deer hunting as my primary example of fun and the need for people to do more of what they love to do, I actually used "going fishing" as my mantra for having them incorporate a will to live in their daily routine.

When I first moved to Pennsylvania after completing my doctorate degree, I lived just outside of State College in a little township called Fisherman's Paradise. Directly behind my house was Spring Creek, the longest, best-known trout stream in Pennsylvania. No matter what the weather, I swear there were always people fly-fishing in this stream. I could see them easily from my back deck. It was such a serene image. This sense that I had about people fully immersed in doing what they loved was epitomized by this image of fly-fishing. The image evoked thoughts and feelings of joy, bliss, and peace, where nothing else mattered. So, very quickly, as part of my promoting a will to live, I told people to go fishing. Of course this didn't have to literally mean fishing or deer hunting. It meant to do whatever brought them the greatest joy and meaning.

This was becoming more and more logical and meaningful for them and for me. It was perfectly aligned with what Dr. Joseph Campbell found to be an ages-old philosophy and wisdom, "Follow your bliss." It also was the message, of course, of Larry LeShan and Carl Simonton, who had considerable clinical experience teaching and encouraging cancer patients and their families to find their own unique song to sing and being more of who they really are, and that took them in the direction of their greatest joy.

While Larry and Carl were the early bandleaders for this message, a cancer surgeon named Bernie Siegel wrote a book titled, *Love, Medicine and Miracles* in 1986.

It became the most widely read book on psychosocial cancer care promoting the role of the will to live, the power of the mind, and that people can work to heal themselves. The popularity of Bernie's message was very distressing to the medical community. The good news is that it stirred research to attempt to prove that this was quackery and giving people false hope. But in fact, major research in 1989 and 1990 supported the role of supportive group therapy and psychoeducational approaches. Other books were appearing, also documenting more scientific evidence for the role of psychosocial factors affecting cancer. Some that I referenced in my classes included: *Behavior and Cancer: Life-Style and Psychological Factors in the Initiation and Progression of Cancer* (1985) by Dr. Sandra M. Levy; *Minding the Body, Mending the Mind* (1987) by Dr. Joan Borysenko; *Head First: The Biology of Hope* (1989) by Norman Cousins; *Cancer as a Turning Point* (1989) by Dr. Lawrence LeShan; and *The Type C Connection: The Behavioral Links to Cancer and Your Health* (1992) by Dr. Lydia Temoshok and Henry Dreher.

It's Too Selfish

But I was in for another surprise. No matter how much common sense and research I gave patients, stating that a strong will to live could affect their health, they thought that taking time for themselves to do what gave them the greatest enthusiasm for life was too selfish. Their moral, social, and cultural conditioning taught them that everyone and everything else should come first. I found that there's a strong tendency for people to believe that doing for others is much more appropriate than creating a balance between taking care of themselves (that's the selfish part) and taking care of others. It was more appropriate to work than to play. I soon realized that I had to give them another "dose" of common sense to help them rethink this position.

Following up on my story about the merits of deer hunting, I began to tell people about how my Dad only ever had at most two weeks of vacation time from work each year. And, of course, one of the weeks was always used for the first week of buck season. It was a given that Dad went hunting with my Uncle Henry every year for one of his total of two weeks of vacation. It never occurred to us to ask him to do something else. We all accepted that ipso facto. An interesting question, however, is, "What would my mother have had to go through if she wanted to disappear for a week?" The real question, of course, was, "Who made this stuff up?" This led to some interesting discussions in our classes and a greater rationale for really thinking about one's individual interests, needs, and values, and the appropriateness of getting these met.

I was finding it an interesting challenge to support these people as they opened to realizing that they had greater choices in their lives than they had imagined. I also felt very honored that they were willing to trust me enough to give me a chance to help them in this way, especially since it forced them to rethink some long-standing, strongly-held ideas about themselves, life, and their health.

When I was in my doctoral program, part of our training was to work in the university counseling center. I often found that students chose a field of study, and assumed it would suit them. I learned that I needed to help them discover more about who they were, and then to identify a career that suited their individual make-up. We then began to list and consider their unique interests, needs, and values.

This university experience enabled me to help my cancer patients appreciate the need to identify and address what mattered most to them. When I asked them to think about their needs, some of the women in particular, really struggled with this. Their primary role and focus in life was on their marriage and family. And, of course, everyone else came first. So, I tried to explain that one way or another they were going to get their needs met. I told them that they needed to get their needs met appropriately or that they would end up getting them met inappropriately. I explain this in detail in my book, *Doctor's Orders: Go Fishing.*

Getting your needs met inappropriately is what is meant regarding the "secondary gains" of illness. People's illness, including cancer, can have secondary gains, which may directly contribute to the onset or duration of the medical condition. I remember at the Simonton Cancer Center being surprised at first when Carl would ask patients, "What is a benefit of cancer? What important needs are being met through your having cancer?" And a common answer was that cancer allowed them to say, "No."

This reminded me of a study with AIDS patients. Often when we study illness, we try to figure out why people got sick instead of looking at people who have done well and why they're healthier. In this AIDS study, they took a group of patients who had fared much better than the norm, and wondered if there were any psychological factors that could explain why they were healthier. The only factor that stood out was that the group who was doing better had a greater ability to say, "No." "Can you refuse an unwanted favor?" was the only question that predicted a better outcome. This was related to a general belief: "I'm worth taking care of." We've learned to try to please others and not meet our own needs.

This helped to strengthen my rationale for not only doing more of what you really want to do, but to do less of what you really don't want to do. So, is it selfish to think about and make an effort to meet your needs? Or is it good sense and another way to improve your health?

<u>Taking Control Of Your Health</u>

I called the program that I developed and taught for these cancer centers, "Taking Control of Your Health". It met for two hours each week for six weeks. The first class covered the "will to live" and the need to "go fishing." I also introduced guided imagery as a tool to reinforce the ideas of each class. People were given an audiocassette of six guided imagery exercises that I had written and recorded for this purpose. They were to listen to one of them daily, especially to support the information presented for that week's class.

Guided imagery is actually a form of mental rehearsal. It is the mental picturing, or sensing, thinking and feeling of a desired outcome. In the same way that you can learn something by practicing or observing, you can learn by imitating this behavior or outcome through thought and imagination. It's like daydreaming on purpose. It draws heavily on the placebo effect, which is based on your beliefs and expectations.

In actual practice, hypnosis and guided imagery are very similar. Hypnosis relies on your expectation and acceptance of a suggestion. So, I had people imagine and accept that: 1) their immune system functioned properly eliminating cancer cells, 2) that they responded well to their medical treatments, and 3) they now felt relaxed, hopeful, and had a renewed enthusiasm for life. These images and suggestions, along with their positive feelings, would act to create these very outcomes.

The second class focused on related mental relaxation techniques, including meditation, mindfulness, prayer, autogenic training, progressive relaxation, systematic desensitization, biofeedback, more information regarding hypnosis and guided imagery, and the power of the mind to affect the body. I also introduced the research in psychoneuroimmunology, which demonstrated the interaction between the central nervous and immune systems. I taught them how you could regulate the immune system through classical conditioning, a form of learning. And how your emotional state directly affected the effectiveness of your immune system.

I also covered the importance of nutrition and exercise. I cited Dr. Andrew Weil and the research by cardiologist, Dr. Dean Ornish, who deserves the highest accolades for proving that you can reverse heart disease with a program of proper nutrition, exercise, and stress management.

In my third class I taught approaches to stress management and how stress affects the way the body fights disease. Class #4 was about how to overcome childhood conditioning and low self-esteem. Here I also raised the question, "Who are you?" (We are mental, emotional, and spiritual: more than our physical bodies).

This is where I introduced love and compassion as a way to deal with suffering, although it wasn't until 1994 that I got hooked on why love heals. Class #5 involved how to develop creativity and intuition. And class #6 was a discussion of goal setting, including one's interests, needs, values, feelings, social support, nutrition, exercise, mental relaxation techniques, fun, and life purpose.

Research Confirmation

I wanted to quickly review for you what I had included in my six-week program so that you might appreciate the outcome of my research looking at the effectiveness of these twelve hours of education. While Carl Simonton and I were aware that this approach had the potential to extend life with cancer, we were very focused on people's quality of life (and quality of death). Of course we were thrilled to find that my research confirmed Carl's findings that this psychosocial approach could affect survival with cancer.

I've mentioned that I lived near State College, Pennsylvania. This is where the offices for the physician management group of cancer centers were based. This also is where Penn State University is located. At some point during my teaching my classes for these cancer centers I met Dr. Ray Palmer, an epidemiologist in the Biobehavioral Health Department at Penn State. He was genuinely interested in the content of my program and proposed a way we could measure its effectiveness.

We compared patients who had been through the program at least four years with matched controls from the same hospitals. We asked tumor registrars in the three cancer centers/hospitals where the program had been

offered most extensively to find patients who had the
same type and stage of cancer to compare to the cancer
patients in our program. They were also matched on age,
date of diagnosis, age at diagnosis, gender, and types of
medical treatment. We found two or three very close
matches for 50 patients who had stage 1 breast or prostate
cancer. There were not enough patients with other than
stage 1 breast or prostate cancer to analyze statistically
and include in the study. In the final analysis, 21 stage 1
breast cancer women and 29 stage 1 prostate cancer men
were compared to 74 and 65 matched patients. The details
of the study were published in May 1999 in the journal,
Alternative Therapies In Health and Medicine. The results
were that the intervention group lived significantly longer
than did their matched-controls. At four to seven years
follow-up (median = 4.2 years), none of the breast cancer
patients in the intervention group died, while 12% of the
control group died. Twice as many of the matched-control
prostate cancer patients died compared to the intervention
group, 28% vs. 14%.

Dr. Larry Dossey was the executive editor of the
journal, *Alternative Therapies in Health and Medicine*,
and Dr. Jeanne Achterberg was the senior editor. I was
very flattered when Jeanne and her husband, Dr. Frank
Lawliss, reviewed the research and recommended to
Larry to publish the results. I had admired the work of
Jeanne and Larry for many years, so I was very pleased to
have them ask to publish the research. And this brought
its own surprises.

When you publish research you must support your
"results" and "discussion" with other existing primary
research findings. It almost never is acceptable to discuss
your clinical, subjective observations as part of why the

treatment was effective. However, Jeanne told me that people are going to want to know why twelve hours of instruction could affect survival with cancer. She wanted me to elaborate and to pose hypotheses, "even speculatively," as to how such a relatively short intervention could result in such large changes in survival rates.

As part of this "speculation" I remarked in the journal "that our patients believed that our program helped them not because of any specific coping skill they learned, but because they felt listened to, cared for, supported, and a sense of connectedness within the group." The reason I wrote this was based on another major surprise I had in working with these cancer centers.

Chapter 3 - To Feel Loved And Cared For

My responsibility as Director of Mind-Body Medicine was to develop all psychological services for cancer patients and their families. It was a FULL-TIME job. I usually drove to four, and sometimes five, cancer centers every week to be available to assist cancer patients and their families. I was there when their radiation treatments began by seven or eight o'clock in the morning, and stayed to teach my two-hour program in the evening, usually six to eight o'clock. Then I drove back home or on to the next cancer center with a similar twelve-hour-plus day.

There were far more cancer centers than I could handle myself. I had a core of three centers that I went to for several years. These were located in State College, Lewistown, and Pottsville, Pennsylvania. But I also taught my classes in other centers in Pennsylvania, as well as traveling to teach in Ohio, New York, and Maryland. Obviously, it was impossible for me to get to all of these centers each week. What helped me was that eventually all of the centers had computers and monitors where the physicians could share X-rays. I then was able to use this technology to reach many more of these centers through video teleconferencing.

However, before I could teleconference, I needed to teach the program myself while we were assessing its effectiveness and trying to find others to help me deliver these psychological services. So, after teaching my classes weekly in Indiana, Pennsylvania for a full year, I then was able to have someone else come in to take my place while I moved on to help at another center. I had gotten to know these patients very well, and I asked them for feedback about the classes. I explained that I had a pretty good idea about what I wanted to teach and why I believed it could help them. But now I wanted to know, of all the things I taught them, what helped them the most, and what didn't. Their feedback would be valuable as I worked at other centers, giving me information on what I could modify or change based on their experience.

The first thing they said that helped them the most was that I listened. I can't tell you how confused I was by this response! My perception of myself was that I taught; I didn't listen. I was sure that they didn't understand my question, so I asked again, "What of all the things I taught in the six classes helped you the most, and what didn't?"

The second thing they said that they learned that helped them was that I cared. Now I was not only confused, but also found myself becoming upset that they obviously didn't understand my question. So, this time I went over all of the six classes in detail, asking and expecting them to say that what helped them was guided imagery, the will to live or "going fishing," stress management, etc. The third thing they now said that helped them the most was that I was sincere.

Believe it or not, I finally started to get it. What helped them the most was not any specific coping skill, but that they felt listened to and cared for.

I must admit that I truly was slow to understand that what I said or taught was not as effective in helping them as the heartfelt way I said it. While I didn't realize this at the time, this experience was pivotal in guiding me to learn and question why love heals. I will talk next in more detail about the healing benefits of heartfelt communication, but I was now learning first-hand that when people feel heard and understood, that this intimate connection is far more meaningful than I had ever thought possible.

When I wrote my research article, I cited one study in particular, by Berland, to support my finding that these psychosocial factors could contribute to survival. In this research, Berland says:

> ...cancer patients who survived many years longer than their "terminal" medical prognoses gave almost twice the credit for their recovery to factors other than their medical treatment. These factors included spiritual, attitudinal, and behavioral attributes (including support of family and friends, individual and group therapy, visualization [guided imagery], and God.

Loneliness and Isolation

I learned long after I published my research that the role of social support, communication and listening had been given decided support from psychologist, Dr. James Lynch. His more than thirty years of research has demonstrated that people's cardiovascular and neuromuscular systems are directly affected by their communication. Blood pressure rises (within 30 seconds) almost always 10-50% when people begin to speak. This is true for all people, healthy and unhealthy (except for schizophrenics). Blood pressure surges are greater while talking than when walking on a treadmill at maximal capacity! However, blood pressure drops rapidly when listening to others in a non-defensive way. This held true for deaf mutes using sign language, also. Their blood pressure increased just like all others, suggesting that it is not talking per se, but the act of communicating that's vital. The key here is that when people feel heard and understood, their bodies respond in a far healthier way than when the conversation is not "heartfelt".

When people speak without "heart", without any real feelings of connection to another, the cardiovascular data are very clear: They are at much higher risk for heart disease and premature death. Dr. Lynch believes that love and felt dialogue are essential for good health. His research determined that loneliness and chronic lack of heartfelt human dialogue were linked to hypertension (high blood pressure) and heart disease. When people do not, or are unable to speak from their heart, their health is at risk!

Dr. Lynch's 1978 book, *The Broken Heart: The Medical Consequences of Loneliness*, was the first to demonstrate how loneliness contributed to all forms of premature death, especially from heart disease. His 1985 book, *The Language of the Heart: The Body's Response to Human Dialogue*, and his 2000 book, *A Cry Unheard: New Insights into the Medical Consequences of Loneliness*, document and describe how loneliness remains an unrecognized and critical medical danger. He concludes that people will search (unconsciously), to the point of physical exhaustion (death), to feel loved and understood. This research supports so clearly why love heals.

Before I go on, I want to stress here what I think is extra important about Dr. Lynch's extensive research demonstrating the need for heartfelt communication. When I was conducting my research for my doctoral dissertation, I was highly trained in research design and the need to control for any variables that might contaminate the research. In my dissertation I tested the effectiveness of Dr. Herbert Benson's relaxation response technique compared to relaxation with specific guided imagery, and to a no-treatment control group. The conclusion was that neither the relaxation response technique nor guided imagery were effective treatments. In fact, the control group often out-performed the treatments.

In the formal "Discussion" of my dissertation, I attempted to explain the results of the research. I wrote, "Due to the guidelines required in introducing this research project to the students, they were not informed of the potential consequences/benefits of the treatments…" I was not allowed to do or say anything that might bias the treatments in any way. I had to remain neutral and, really, quite mechanical. There was no heartfelt communication with the students who participated in the study. It was all so unnatural.

This leads me to a comment I want to make regarding what Dr. Dean Ornish said was one of the single best studies for proving that the mind is involved in physical health. In 1989 psychiatrist David Spiegel and colleagues at Stanford Medical School conducted research to *disprove* that psychosocial interventions could affect survival with cancer. In this well designed, randomized study, women with breast cancer met weekly in a support group for one year. The outcome was that they lived twice as long as did the other breast cancer patients who didn't have the support group!

In a 1989 article in the journal, *Advances in Mind-Body Medicine*, Ornish wrote that this clearly demonstrated "the need for social support, community, and intimacy...integral to our survival." He noted that as a result of the weekly support group sessions, "a strong sense of community and intimacy developed."

This study headed by Dr. Spiegel was replicated and published in 2001 in the *New England Journal of Medicine*. Here, Dr. P. J. Goodwin and colleagues at the University of Toronto followed Dr. Spiegel's protocol, and even had Dr. Spiegel consult on the study to be sure it was a true replication of his original research. Goodwin's study, however, concluded, "Supportive-expressive group therapy does not prolong survival in women with metastatic breast cancer."

I attended a conference soon after the publication of Goodwin's research, where both Dr. Goodwin and Dr. Spiegel made presentations. We in the audience were a bit baffled at the distinctly different outcomes. This brings me to the question I really want to raise. Was the Goodwin study so stringently conducted, in order to truly replicate Spiegel's research, that it lacked the same heartfelt connection that developed in the Stanford support group?

This illustrates a complexing issue in conducting any mind-body research. Even in the most rigorously controlled, randomized studies, it is very difficult to control for all of the human factors. I can't help but wonder about the quality of any research or the effectiveness of any psychosocial treatment that does not include the role of intimacy and heartfelt communication, where people feel truly heard and understood.

When I was developing the content of the program I taught at the cancer centers, I was very much aware of the research and potential benefit of social support and support groups. I assumed that the classes I taught could and would serve as an opportunity for cancer patients and their families to socialize and support each other. The last thing I wanted for them was to withdraw from life and wait to die. Remember: I wanted them to go fishing! But they didn't – not enough for me to confidently conclude that this is why they lived longer. This is when I came to really value the research and insights of Dr. Dean Ornish.

I once read an article where it asked several noted health professionals to name the one scientific study that has contributed most to our understanding of health and medicine. If I had been asked, it would be Dean Ornish and his colleagues' research published in 1995 in the *Journal of the American Medical Association*. They found that patients diagnosed with heart disease could stop or begin to reverse the disease following lifestyle changes in nutrition, physical exercise, and stress management. And that even severe coronary heart disease often begins to reverse when making these lifestyle changes, without drugs or surgery. His book, *Dr. Dean Ornish's Program for Reversing Heart Disease*, was the best comprehensive approach to health I'd ever read. And his book, *Love and Survival*, was the icing on the cake.

To this day, when people think or talk about Ornish's research and program, they focus primarily on the role of nutrition. Although many consider his low fat, vegetarian diet relatively extreme, his research showed that those patients who adhered most strictly to this diet fared better than those who didn't in reversing their heart disease. However, Ornish wrote extensively in his books that he believed it was the stress management component that was the greatest factor in the reversal of their disease.

The stress management techniques in his "Opening Your Heart Program" included a comprehensive practice of yoga, (stretching exercises, progressive relaxation, breathing techniques, meditation, and guided and receptive imagery), communication skills, and other techniques for creating intimacy. Dr. Ornish had studied and practiced these stress management techniques derived from yoga, and believed that they addressed the more fundamental issues that predispose people to illness. All of these techniques or methods had a common purpose: to heal people's isolation.

A recurrent theme in his book and program for reversing heart disease is that:

> ...Isolation can lead to stress and, ultimately, to illness, whereas intimacy can be healing. Isolation comes in several forms:
>
> • Isolation from our feelings, our inner self, and inner peace
> • Isolation from others
> • Isolation from a higher force

In 1998 Dr. Dean Ornish published *Love and Survival*, where he cited considerable compelling research documenting the healing benefits of love. After 20 years of research and practice, he wrote in italics, *"I am not aware of any other factor in medicine – not diet, not smoking, not exercise, not stress, not genetics, not drugs, not surgery – that has a greater impact on our quality of life, incidence of illness, and premature death from of all causes"* than the role of love and intimacy.

Dr. Ornish wrote further that social and emotional support relate to a common theme: "When you feel loved, nurtured, cared for, supported, and intimate, you are much more likely to be happier and healthier. You have a much lower risk of getting sick, and, if you do, a much greater chance of surviving." Whatever words or terms people use scientifically to explain the role of social support, he believes it all comes down to, "Do you feel loved and cared for?"

It is very clear from the extensive research of Dr. James Lynch and Dr. Dean Ornish that feeling heard, understood, loved, and cared for are major factors in healing. And I have to agree. It's been almost ten years since I published my research with cancer patients where I concluded that the reason they lived longer was "because they felt listened to, cared for, supported, and a sense of connectedness within the group." Nothing has happened since to change my mind, and, in fact, I am that much more certain about the healing power of feeling loved, which is what has driven me to write this book.

Why Suffering?

Before I began my work with cancer, I worked as a staff psychologist for a rehabilitation hospital, as I mentioned earlier. People were admitted to the hospital primarily because they had a stroke. I remember, at first, feeling quite confident, and telling patients and families that everything would be all right, that it was just a matter of time and appropriate treatment. I was in for another surprise.

While most of these patients fared relatively well, it often was a longer and more arduous process than I imagined. Not only was their treatment difficult (patients came to call their physical therapy "licensed torture"), but there was far more emotional pain and suffering than I was prepared for. Soon, instead of feeling confident about my role in helping them, I found myself too often feeling helpless.

Patients had a huge adjustment to make from having a very independent lifestyle, to now having up to half their body paralyzed. Families were forced into the role of caregivers, having to change their lives almost completely, which they often resented. This usually included their questioning their spiritual faith. How could God let this happen?

This experience led me to numbers of questions like, Why suffering? Does life serve a purpose? And if it does, then why suffering? If there is an all-knowing and all-loving God, if this is a benevolent universe, then what is the role of suffering? Not only did I want to understand suffering so that I could be of greater help to people, but it was important for my own personal understanding, as well.

I grew up thinking that suffering was a form of spiritual punishment. In my religious training, I was taught that God was loving, but that God also could be vengeful. If you didn't obey God's will, you would go to hell and burn for eternity.

Eventually I found myself reading more philosophical books and articles that addressed the subject of suffering. It seemed that suffering forced people to question "Why?" or "Why me?" Perhaps as much as any other question, suffering caused people to look at what they really believe. As I began to investigate religious and spiritual belief systems, and what they had to say about suffering, I was not surprised to find that they disagreed considerably regarding what was necessary for enlightenment or to follow and fulfill God's will. What did surprise me is that they managed to agree on two major points: 1) that we are all one with God, and 2) that there is a common moral code, the Golden Rule.

Every major religion has attempted to explain the ultimate nature of reality and has advised people how to live. Hinduism, Buddhism, Taoism, Judaism, Christianity, and Islam have all taught that there is an ultimate source of all being, which is omnipresent in all things, and that we are one with everything. And each religion has taught a form of the Golden Rule: Do unto others, as you would have them do unto you. The ultimate purpose in life is to realize the Eternal Self within, to know of one's union with God or a Divine Source, and ways to live in harmony with all of creation.

Since then I have read and learned more about the common beliefs of major religious and philosophical groups, which I'll address later. But asking these big questions about the role of suffering, and does life serve a purpose, kept bringing me back to one point: the consideration of love.

The Purpose of Life

You'll remember that my great friend and mentor, Ken McCaulley, had been a genuine seeker of Truth. And as part of his life path he became an ordained Presbyterian minister, earned a doctorate degree in metaphysics, and meditated daily for years. He taught me that the purpose of life was related to learning to love.

He cited how, in the New Testament, (Matthew 22:36-40), Jesus was asked:

> "Teacher, which is the greatest commandment in the law?" Jesus replied, "Love the Lord your God with all your heart and with all your soul and with all your mind. This is the first and greatest commandment. And the second is like it: Love your neighbor as yourself. All the laws and prophets hang on these two commandments."

I remember how surprised I was that this was all Jesus had to say in his answer. He seemed to have left out quite a lot according to my religious training.

As I mentioned, Ken was indeed a scholar. He had studied Greek and Aramaic, and had read the earliest, closet copies of the original Bible. In fact, he told me there is no original Bible. The closest copy is a tertiary source: a copy of a copy of a copy. He knew that much of the Bible had been transliterated, misinterpreted, miscopied, or purposefully distorted to support religious groups wanting to monopolize authority.

Ken recommended that I read Norman Cousins' book, *In God We Trust: The Religious Beliefs and Ideals of the American Founding Fathers*, where he discussed how most of the founding fathers resisted many of the beliefs of the Bible. They believed that Jesus' moral teachings were sound principles, but that they were likely corrupted and changed throughout history by groups and governments seeking power.

President Thomas Jefferson was a very outspoken critic of religion. In his book, *The Life and Morals of Jesus*, Jefferson extracted all of the unloving sayings, stories and acts attributed to Jesus. He condensed the New Testament into a rather small book containing only Jesus' loving words and acts, which has come to be known as the Jefferson Bible. Jefferson believed that Christianity was "the most sublime and benevolent" philosophy ever created, and yet "the most perverted".

Although my friend Ken had entered the ministry in his search for truth, he eventually left the church because he felt that its dogma had gotten too far from teaching love and how to apply it in our daily lives. This is when he began many years of daily meditation, which led to his developing his own self-improvement program, which emphasized the importance of "manifesting love".

As I mentioned in the first chapter of this book, soon after I met Ken, we began to meditate together. We connected daily with what we called "mentors", or some might call "spiritual guides". We were constantly reminded by these guides that the primary purpose of life was to learn and demonstrate love.

This coincided with the research of Dr. Raymond Moody. In his book, *Life after Life*, he described a common scenario for people who have had a near death experience. People who are clinically dead and then return to life often report an experience of being separate from their bodies before coming into the presence of an overwhelming light. This light is experienced as the most intense feeling of love and acceptance. People tend to interpret this light as the presence of God or some spiritual being related to their earthly religious experience. As part of their life review, people are asked by this Supreme Being of Light two basic questions: "Have you learned to love?" and "Are you satisfied with what you've learned?" To learn to love appeared to be the purpose for human existence according to Dr. Moody and his research with near death experiences.

As I thought more about the possibility that life served the purpose of learning to love, I found myself asking the question: When we got to the end of our physical life, how would we know whether or not we had learned to love? Would we add up the number of times we hugged or kissed someone? Would we have to have a certain number of good deeds? I asked these questions in earnest, and I found that I really wasn't sure what it meant to love.

In my scientific training I was taught that in order to measure something you had to define it first. And in order to do that, sometimes you had to give it an "operational" definition. What objective evidence was there to measure whether or not something happened? If we were trying to measure or observe love, what behaviors would define and indicate that someone was demonstrating loving behavior?

I reflected on my Christian religious training and remembered when the prophet Micah (6:8) spoke of what the Lord required: "To act justly and to love mercy and to walk humbly with your God." The apostle Paul talked about the importance of faith, hope, and charity. I thought about Jesus and the qualities and character of his person. I also remembered my Boy Scout training and that one was to be thrifty, brave, reverent, etc. I thought that these would be examples of loving behavior; that is, if one were just or fair, merciful, humble, charitable, and reverent, these would be demonstrations of love.

I thought of other qualities or traits that similarly would demonstrate love: compassion, kindness, caring, listening, sensitivity, support, tenderness, patience, sincerity, loyalty, friendship, sympathy, respect, courage etc. Then it occurred to me that these were the very qualities or behaviors that we usually admire most, especially at a time of crisis. I thought about patients and families who had strokes, or great pain and upset, and how the experience of suffering and distress could teach us the real value of love. It is when we are feeling most travailed that we truly learn to appreciate loving acts.

If life serves the purpose of learning to love, times of suffering may actually be blessings in disguise! This doesn't mean that suffering is necessary or that it is the only or best way to learn to love. Metaphysicians have referred to human existence as "a veil of tears." It seems to be a given that life is going to have its turmoil. However, if life is about learning to love, then human existence with all of it's seeming tragedy and suffering, may be just what the doctor ordered.

The Four Noble Truths of Buddhism deal with the inevitable fact of suffering. Life is suffering. A fundamental practice for Buddhists is to pray with thanks for their illness, crisis, or suffering for aiding their spiritual growth. In his book, *A Path With Heart*, Jack Kornfield talks about his training and experience as a Buddhist monk. One chapter is titled, "Turning Straw Into Gold."

Like the young maiden in the fairy
tale "Rumpelstiltskin" who is locked in a

room full of straw, we often do not realize that the straw all around us is gold in disguise. The basic principle of spiritual life is that our problems become the very place to discover wisdom and love.

Other books like *Minding the Body, Mending the Mind* by Joan Borysenko; Man's *Search for Meaning* by Viktor Frankl; and *The Healing Family* by Stephanie Simonton helped me in my understanding of a rationale for suffering as a part of life. But it was in 1993 and 1994 that I really came to deeply understand that spirituality and love are significant factors in health and healing.

Love Heals

In 1993, there were two excellent mind-body health videos produced and aired on television. The first was Bill Moyers' *Healing and the Mind*, televised by PBS. The second was *The Heart of Healing*, televised by TBS. Both were documentaries discussing "alternative" approaches to healthcare throughout the world.

Bill Moyers' video begins with an interview in China with Dr. David Eisenberg, a Harvard medical doctor. Dr. Eisenberg headed the study of the use of unconventional medicine in the United States published in the *New England Journal of Medicine* in 1993. He reported that people in 1990 were going to "alternative" practitioners more than their primary care physicians for their health care. This has become the most cited medical journal article in history. Dr. Eisenberg replicated this survey in 1997, and published it in the *Journal of the American Medical Association* in 1998. The survey concluded that alternative medicine use has increased substantially between 1990 and 1997. Bill Moyers' video is an excellent documentary of these alternative medical therapies and how the mind affects the body.

The Heart of Healing video is a similar documentary about mind-body health. It's how people around the world described their use of alternative therapies, which they believed healed them. In one segment of this video, Roger Pilon, MD, Director of the Medical Bureau Lourdes, is discussing miracles. Miracles are a controversial subject for science since they imply a suspension of law. The Catholic Church, under very strict criteria, has declared 65 people to have had a miracle. When Dr. Pilon was asked why he believed these people overcame their incurable illnesses, he proposed, "They had faith in someone who loves us."

I was quite taken by this response. The idea of faith and the placebo effect was not new to me at all, but the role of love surprised me coming from a highly respected medical doctor. I remember I was compelled to keep watching the video.

In the next scene Father Henri Joulia of the Sanctuary of Notre Dame of Lourdes was asked, in a totally separate interview, the same question, "Why did these people have a miracle?" Father Joulia responded, "They had a sense of being loved and cared for." They knew that they were loved unconditionally; "God loves *me!*" "God loves *me!*"

Once more I was taken by the consideration of love as the reason for their cure. When I thought about this more academically I, again, understood how one's belief could make a difference. I knew also of the strong role that social support can play. But I found myself very caught up in the idea that when someone felt completely loved that it could affect such dramatic healing. This idea stayed with me for months.

Then one day in the Spring of 1994 I was watching the Oprah Winfrey Show on television. She was interviewing Maya Angelou, the wonderful poet and orator. I have never heard a better speaker than Maya Angelou, and she always speaks from the depth of her soul.

Oprah was being her very Oprah self, very personable, genuine, and friendly. She asked Maya what it was like to get a phone call from the White House asking her to write and deliver the poem for President Clinton's January, 1993, Inaugural Ceremony. Maya told her, "My knees started to turn to water." When Oprah asked her if she felt any pressure, Maya said, "What allows me to go from darkness into darkness is a profound faith. I am a child of God." She said this with remarkable confidence and clarity.

Maya then sang a line from a 19th century spiritual song, "I don't believe he brought me this far to leave me." And, again, with great clarity, Maya said, "I know that I'm a child of God," and "I'm up to it" [writing and delivering the poem]. "I come from the Creator like everybody else trailing wisps of glory." She continued, "I gave my energy to God and said if this is what you want done, I will do it."

When Oprah asked Maya if this was one of her proudest moments, Maya replied, "Sometimes people think that the public recognition's the greatest thing that can happen." But Maya proposed, "Some private revelations can be greater." Maya then reflected back to 1953 when a voice and spiritual teacher taught her, "God loves *me*!" Maya thought that this was one of the greatest moments in her life, the knowing that "God loves *me*…and when you *know* it…I can do anything I want to do. I can do it." To this day, whenever Maya repeats to herself "God loves me," she is "filled with wonder" knowing that God loves her unconditionally, the "good" and the "bad."

I could never duplicate in writing about this interview the depth of feeling Maya brought to these words "God loves me." It clearly moved Oprah Winfrey, also. Oprah ended her show with the statement, "The greatest thing I learned which I'm going to take with me is, God loves me." And I cannot express fully enough now how deeply moved I was, too.

This was a special moment for me for another reason. It "clicked" for me that, indeed, people could be healed when they knew God loved them. It was a deep realization of who they really are – a part of God. This is who I am! "As it was in the beginning, is now and ever shall be." I am one with God. Not only does God love me unconditionally, but this is who I am.

What I found in teaching my classes was that the one thing we're all looking for is peace of mind. And you get peace of mind when you're truly being yourself. Now it occurred to me: that at the deepest level, you are most yourself when you realize your oneness with God! I will discuss this at length in the next chapter. But firstly I feel it's important to raise the question, "What is love?"

What Is Love?

Based on my research and experience in teaching cancer patients and their families about a psychosocial approach to cancer care, I came to conclude, like Dean Ornish, that feeling loved and cared for was in fact a major factor in health and healing. I found James Lynch's work and research to be outstanding support for this conclusion as well. This is what led me to really believe why love heals. But before I introduce other evidence, I think it's appropriate to attempt to define what love is (beyond my earlier initial operational definition of love).

When I was writing *Doctor's Orders: Go Fishing*, I was reminded constantly (intuitively) that nothing heals like love and tenderness. This idea isn't exactly new. We're all familiar with the expression TLC, tender loving care. Nurses, in particular, were noted for administering TLC as part of their standard of care. For all of the above reasons, we could say that love includes feeling cared for, listened to, and understood.

Character Strengths and Virtues

In preparation for this book, I read *Character Strengths and Virtues* by Dr. Christopher Peterson and Dr. Martin Seligman. This almost 800 page academic handbook is a very worthy manual of psychological health. Where the Diagnostic and Statistical Manual of Mental Disorders (DSM) is used by all mental health professionals and physicians to diagnose mental disorders, its focus is on illness, not health. Peterson and Seligman propose that we need to focus on what is right with people, not what is wrong, and they developed a classification of character strengths and virtues. After reviewing all of the philosophic and scientific literature, they discovered six broad core characteristics of virtue: wisdom, courage, humanity, justice, temperance, and transcendence. "We argue that these are universal, perhaps grounded in biology through an evolutionary process that selected for these aspects of excellence as means of solving the important tasks for survival of the species."

The authors concentrated on the dominant spiritual and philosophical traditions of Confucianism and Taoism in China, Buddhism and Hinduism in South Asia, ancient Greece, Judo-Christianity, and Islam in the West. Their review revealed scientifically measurable cognitive, behavioral, and emotional traits and experiences that supported the character strengths within these virtues.

Character strengths are the psychological ingredients that define the virtues. Love is listed as a character strength within the virtue of humanity, which is generally defined as caring relationships with others. Love included the sharing of aid, comfort, and acceptance. "It involves strong positive feelings, commitment, and even sacrifice."

I am very grateful for this extensive, overwhelming survey that found these virtues and strengths to be so ubiquitous and universally valued. It helps me appreciate more the value and purpose of philosophical and spiritual systems and religions.

My early life experience with religion focused on beliefs and dogma over the development of character strengths and virtues. This was Ken's experience as a Presbyterian minister, and the reason why he left the church. Religions, at their best, are teaching people how to develop personal character traits, which will help them survive and prosper. Ken's belief was that they should be teaching how to manifest love – the consensus purpose of life itself.

Peterson and Seligman's classification of character strengths and virtues, and their promotion of happiness and fulfillment, certainly adds an academic understanding of what love is. We could easily include every character strength and virtue within an operational definition of love. Peterson's and Seligman's complete list include:

1. Wisdom and knowledge (creativity, curiosity/love of learning, open-mindedness, perspective)
2. Courage (bravery, persistence, integrity, vitality)
3. Humanity (love, kindness, social intelligence)
4. Justice (citizenship, fairness, leadership)
5. Temperance (forgiveness, mercy, humility, modesty, prudence, moderation, self-regulation)
6. Transcendence (appreciation of beauty, gratitude, hope, humor, spirituality)

Qualities of generosity, nurturance, care, compassion, altruistic love, and niceness are included within the character strength of kindness. I think that these are what most people think of if attempting to define love. Most commonly, I've thought of love as a deep caring for and acceptance of oneself and others just the way we are. In a word, I could define love as compassion. In two words, harmonious action. But I want to propose that love is really oneness, and this is why love heals.

Chapter 4 - Oneness

On the cover of my book, *Doctor's Orders: Go Fishing*, I wrote very clearly, "Joy and peace of mind are essential for your health." I believe that joy and peace of mind are two of the greatest aspects of love. Actually, they're very similar. As I've already noted, you have peace of mind most often when you are doing what brings you the greatest joy. And joy, of course, will bring you peace of mind. I'd like to show you one way I learned how they factor into improved health.

One day I was a guest on Dr. Haines Ely's "Earth Mysteries" radio show on KVMR in Nevada City, California, and we were discussing my book and work. I've been his guest numbers of times, and these interviews have always gone very well. When I got home later that day, I received a phone call from a man who had heard the radio show, and wanted very much to meet and talk with me. He told me that he agreed strongly with what I had to say, and wanted to show me a biofeedback device that he had developed. He said it could measure heart coherence or compassion, which for him meant being truly authentic and resonating with your soul. This man's name is James Barrett, and his device is called the Heart Link. We have since become great friends.

I have to be honest and say that much of what he had to say was way over my head. Fortunately, James is very patient with me. A very interesting understanding of his insight into the relationship between the physical and the spiritual can be found in his book, *The Silent Gospel*.

Anyhow, as part of this day of our first meeting he placed two electrodes on my chest near my heart, and showed me on a monitor a moment-to-moment display of my heart rate variability, which appeared as waves or spikes. He explained how these "spikes" would raise in a uniform manner if I were experiencing sustained heart coherence. I practiced guided imagery to relax, and my heart responded accordingly.

Before long we were just chatting away. I had actually forgotten that I was still hooked up to the Heart Link. Then at some point in our conversation James stopped me and wanted me to look at the monitor. He said that I had just registered remarkable heart coherence. Here's why. We were talking about my idea of "going fishing", doing what brought me the greatest joy. And I was talking about spending time with my brothers-in-law. At that time we all loved to eat, drink, smoke cigars, and talk and joke about God-knows-what. We had the greatest time together. And my heart showed it! There was no hiding from my heart the true joy I had when I was with these two.

Heart rate variability is measured by your cardiologist with an electrocardiogram (EKG) to check the health of your heart. The joy I experienced just thinking about times spent with my brothers-in-law were a perfect prescription for my heart! Please understand that I am not recommending gluttony, ample good wine and cigars as a health remedy. But what my soul was mirroring for me was that my heart was singing joyfully. It was happy and healthy. This was my heart and soul's truth, and it showed. For James, this was a perfect demonstration of self-love, of aligning myself with my non-local self or soul. Truth resonates with Truth, is felt as love or oneness, and can be measured as heart coherence. This resonance, this being on the same wave length, this harmony or synchronicity with your heart and soul is what is meant by the experience of oneness.

Meditation

Meditation is an ancient practice for connecting with one's soul. In their book, *Soul Medicine*, Dr. Norman Shealy and Dr. Dawson Church describe it as a shift from our focus on the physical body, thoughts, and circumstances – "to the realm of pure awareness, unmediated by thought." It is a state of consciousness where you experience the blending of your personal soul with the universal soul or God or Divine Source. At this time any perceptions of limitation or separation "are replaced by a state of pervasive peace, and a sense that all is well". Shealy and Dawson state:

> This is the consciousness in which the medicine of the soul may flow into the body. It draws on the power of the universal soul, particularized in the individual soul, to promote healing. It connects with the epigenetic blueprint of healing available at the soul level; at that level, all healing is possible, even miraculous cures. By identifying with that soul level, and the blueprint for health contained at the level, the image of greater perfection can migrate into the concrete physical reality of one's mind, heart, and body.

Meditation usually is associated with Eastern religions, but is in fact a form of prayer associated with all of the major religions including Islam, Judaism, and Christianity. In meditation, it is a common tradition to use the repetition of a word, phrase, or prayer such as in Christianity the repetitious prayer, "Lord Jesus Christ have mercy on me." Meditation is slowly finding its way into medical practice.

Dr. Herbert Benson, an Associate Professor of Medicine at Harvard Medical School, has studied and researched mental relaxation techniques extensively for the past 40 years. At first he studied the effects of transcendental meditation, which included the silent repetition of a sound called a mantra and a passive approach to any distracting thoughts. It was a gentle focusing or narrowing of attention. He found that this approach differed significantly from a normal, quiet, resting state, and also from sleep. By focusing their attention in this way, people were able to decrease their oxygen consumption rate, lower blood lactate levels, produce more low frequency brain waves, lower heart and breathing rate, and decrease muscle tension – all associated with relaxation, the opposite of a stressful response. His 1975 book, *The Relaxation Response*, details much of this early research and this approach which entails, 1) something to focus your attention on which is non-threatening and, ideally, which has meaning for you like a personal affirmation; 2) a quiet environment; 3) a comfortable posture; and 4) a passive attitude. With your eyes closed, this is all meant to focus your attention.

Another form of meditation that has been used with good success in a medical setting is the practice of mindfulness. Dr. Jon Kabat-Zinn has used this mindfulness practice effectively with a broad range of serious physical illnesses. He served as Director of the Stress Reduction Clinic at the University of Massachusetts Medical Center, where he is Professor of Medicine Emeritus. Thousands of people have been referred here by their physicians, usually because more standard medical care has been relatively ineffective with their various health conditions. Interestingly, this program offers the same training in mindfulness and stress reduction to everyone no matter what their diagnosis. Kabat-Zinn explains that his program is a way for people to experience and understand the mind-body connection and to use it to deal more effectively with their life situations. Usually people come with no particular knowledge of meditation or interest in it. But as they learned to acknowledge and be fully present with their stress and pain, they were often able to manage their symptoms more effectively than with conventional medical treatment. You can read about his mindfulness meditation approach in his book, *Full Catastrophe Living*.

Similarly, Dr. Dean Ornish states in his book, *Dr. Dean Ornish's Program for Reversing Heart Disease*, that meditation is a way to manage stress and heart disease:

> …Meditation doesn't smooth out the disturbances in your life, as a tranquilizer might. Meditation allows you to go deeper, to where the disturbances begin. It helps you become more aware of how your mind becomes agitated and gives you more control to stop these disturbances. It doesn't

bring you peace, for the peace is already
there once you stop disturbing it.

Dr. Ornish believes that meditation allows one to
rediscover and begin healing the inner self. Meditation is
a tool for transformation where people can reconnect with
themselves and their feelings, and also spiritually. He
proposes that healing is ultimately healing our sense of
isolation. A common occurrence in meditating is to
experience a connection with something larger than
ourselves, and a deep sense of peace and joy.

When Dr. Martin Rossman and I co-authored the
chapter on Mind-Body Medicine in *Integrative Oncology*
in 2009, we defined meditation as a gentle narrowing and
focusing of one's attention on a neutral or meaningful
subject, such as paying attention to your breathing or a
personal affirmation. In mindfulness meditation you
simply observe whatever thoughts, images, or feelings
that come into your awareness in a passive, nonjudgmental way. The most practical benefit is to still or
quiet the mind, and to refocus your attention on
something other than habitual worries or fears.

An informal practice of mindfulness is really a lot
like the idea, "stop and smell the roses." It may be helpful
here to discuss mindfulness and meditation in this way to
help demystify their concept and practice. When you're
sitting by a fire and watching the flames dance; when
you're sitting on the beach watching the waves roll on
shore; when you're watching a sunset, listening to music,
or doing anything you love in this passive way, this is a
form of meditation.

I'd like to invite you to participate in a meditative
exercise. In this meditation, you seat yourself in a quiet

setting, make yourself comfortable, close your eyes, and ask yourself to feel the energy of your soul. Let yourself receive any sensations, images, words, or feelings that may arise. A spiritual teacher recommended this to me recently. I want to share with you what I experienced. You may experience something totally different, but I was a little surprised by what happened. Here are the images and feelings I had: 1) a white winged horse, which felt like freedom; 2) a fairy princess that felt like feminine magic; 3) a mountain landscape with its majestic beauty; 4) Roman soldiers who felt like a disciplined power; 5) a speed boat with remarkable agility; 6) a cunning, very alert tiger; 7) the grace of a butterfly; 8) the smell and taste of peach cobbler; 9) going on a garden tour and seeing beautiful roses; 10) watching a kitten play with a ball of yarn; 11) a man cutting free and rescuing a whale; 12) an inspiring idea; 13) giving without any thought of anything in return, like inviting someone over for dinner; 14) jousters on horses acknowledging and respecting their opponents before their match; 15) riding a race horse and running free; 16) salt water fish and ducks on a pond with their beautiful colors and markings; 17) the wonder and awe of seeing an elephant or panda; 18) and the rhythm and movement of an ice-skater or ballet dancer. There were times during this exercise when I had the biggest, happiest smile; I almost couldn't contain it. My soul's energy felt curious, impish, and yet wise. It was pure awareness where I felt myself open up, then lift, as if I were floating.

These insights, images, and feelings came from several meditations, but I hope this helps some of you who have little or no experience with meditation to give it a try. In time you will find that it really is a gateway to your soul and Divine Source. The experience can be quite incomparable. It can reveal the truth of who you really are: one with everything. Feeling one with everything is sometimes called a peak, mystical, or transcendent experience, which I discuss in more depth in Chapter 10.

Nature and Weather

You'll remember in Chapter 3 how I found in my investigation of suffering that all religions managed to agree on two things, one of which is that we are all one with God. There is an ultimate source of all being, which is omnipresent in all things, and we are one with that: one with everything. I have to admit that this has been hard for me to really grasp. Doesn't it sound rather grandiose if not psychotic to actually think that this really means that we are God-like. Everything is God manifesting in different form. We are God incarnate. What appears to be separate is all one and the same.

An image that works for me is to think of God as the sun, the eternal Source of life-giving energy. And all life forms are the garden created by the loving, sustaining energy of this all-encompassing Central Sun, which gives growth and creates beauty. While the sun and the garden appear separate, the garden is the Central Sun (God or Divine Consciousness) manifesting as form in an endless act of creation, love and harmony. Flowing through all of creation is the divine radiation of the Central Sun's rays of light. It is who we are. Oneness is the energy or vibration of the Divine Source. And nature is Divine Source in its purest form.

I want to tell a very personal story here to elaborate further on the concept of oneness and nature. When I was developing psychological services for cancer patients, the last thing I wanted was for them to withdraw from life. My big message, of course, was to go fishing: Do what brings you the greatest joy and meaning. So, I decided to have picnics where all patients and their families and friends could get together and have some fun, sponsored by their cancer center. These events soon became very well attended, and truly served my intended purpose.

While they were all quite successful, the ones in Pottsville, Pennsylvania were exceptional, largely due to a man named Bob Hughes. Bob had the biggest heart, almost to a fault. He seemed to know everyone, and he could just make things happen. He lived on a large acreage where he had built a huge pavilion with stoves and refrigerators and everything you could think of to picnic. Beside the pavilion and picnic tables was a pond, which Bob would stock with trout the week before our picnics there. People in the community loved what we were doing, and would donate all kinds of things. The Schuylkill Cancer Center donated the food, and a radio station would even come and do a broadcast from the picnic, encouraging people to come out and join us. No one looked or acted like cancer patients ready to die! I defied media people who came to cover our events to tell me who were the cancer patients.

We usually held these picnics every spring, summer, and fall. And they went on for several years. But what was especially fascinating was that it *never* rained on any of our picnics. It could rain before or after the picnic. It could rain around our picnic. People simply came to know and say to others if there were a threat of rain that might cancel or interfere with the outdoor picnics, "It never rains on our picnics."

I was slow to accept the truth of this because it seemed so strange. What was so special about our events? It was surely coincidence that it didn't rain, but this was in fact the case. However, on Sunday, June 9th, 1996 at Bob Hughes' place, we held our last picnic. I now was going to teach my "Taking Control of Your Health" program through video teleconferencing instead of traveling everywhere and teaching in person. This would allow us to reach many more people in more locations. Toward the end of that afternoon, when I announced to our group that I would not be returning to Pottsville, the skies filled with thunder and lightening, and it poured! God, strike me dead if I'm not telling you the truth.

This had to be coincidence, but it makes a good story, doesn't it? Then many years later I read a book called *Weather Shamanism* by Nan Moss and David Corbin. Anthropologist, Dr. Hank Wesselman, who I knew, wrote a testimonial for the book on the first page stating, "Nan Moss and David Corbin are master shamanic teachers who reveal what becomes possible when we intentionally align ourselves with the ancient forces of nature to alleviate suffering and help restore order when chaos moves in." And on the first page of "Acknowledgments," Nan and David wrote, "Shamanism has always been about partnering with helping spirits." It is the oldest known form of spirituality. Page one of the actual book reads that "we are weather and weather is us." Whether or not we realize it, we are in relationship with weather and nature. Everything is connected, and we affect the weather "*by our psyches and emotions and by our sense of connectedness or disconnectedness from the natural world.*" *Weather Shamanism* concludes that there are those instances in which the weather spirits respond to certain individuals and events "akin to grace."

What I really want to emphasize by telling my story and discussing shamanism is that, "In the shamanic worldview, all that exists is alive, and everything and everyone is interrelated with everything else." Just as I said earlier that everything is God manifesting in different form, weather is Spirit manifesting as rain or clouds or storms. Clouds are real sentient, living beings. I know this might sound odd to many, but wind and rain and clouds and trees and rocks and animals and plants are conscious energy forms, as conscious and responsive to thoughts and emotions as humans. Shamans understand the sacred nature of reality and the oneness of all of life. We are all spirits in different physical forms. We are all part of one divine organism.

Religion

On one level it sounds like blasphemy of the highest order to think of us as one with God. Weren't we taught that God is all goodness and greatness, and we are but His miscreant offspring? Indeed, Jesus had to be sent to save us from our sinful nature. So, how is it that every major religion has also instructed that we are one? Isn't this what it means when we say God is omnipresent? In the Revised Standard Version of the Bible (Ephesians 4:4-6) it states, "There is one body and one Spirit, ...who is above all and through all and in all." In John 14:20, "... I am in my father, and you in me, and I in you." In Matthew 25:40, "Truly, I say to you, as you did it to one of the least of these my brethren, you did it to me." In

Psalms 82:6, "I say, 'you are gods, sons of the Most High, all of you...'"

The book, *Oneness: Great Principles Shared by All Religions*, notes similar statements from other religions. In Hinduism, "the individual soul is nothing else in essence than universal soul." In Islam, "On God's own nature has been molded man's." In Sikhism, "God is concealed in every heart; his light is in every heart."

In the classic book, *The Religions of Man*, Huston Smith surveys the meaning of the worlds' religions. He cites a statement from Zen Buddhism of Japan: "The One is none other than the All, the All none other than the One." Smith claims that no other symbol or statement makes this more clear than the traditional Chinese symbolism of yin and yang, the all embracing circle, symbol of the unity of all of life:

Life does not move onward and upward towards a fixed pinnacle or pole. It turns and bends back upon itself until the self comes full-circle and knows that at center all things are one.

He adds in *Forgotten Truth: The Common Vision of the World's Religions*, "at-one-ment is not a state to be achieved but a condition to be recognized."

Passages from the *Conversations With God* books certainly support our oneness:

This is what your religions mean when they say that you were created in the "image and likeness of God." This doesn't mean, as some have suggested, that our physical bodies look alike (although God can adopt whatever physical form God chooses for a particular purpose.) It does mean that our essence is the same. We are composed of the same stuff. WE ARE the "same stuff." With all the same properties and abilities – including the ability to create physical reality out of thin air.

My purpose in creating you, My Spiritual offspring, was for ME to know Myself as God. I have no way to do that *save through you*. Thus it can be said (and has been, many times) that My purpose for you is that you should know yourself as Me."

In response to a question Neale Donald Walsch, the author of *Conversations With God* book 1, posed to God, God replied:

The promise of God is that you are His son. Her offspring. Its likeness. His equal.

Ah …here is where you get hung up. You can accept "His Son," "offspring," "likeness," but you recoil at being called "His equal". It is too much to accept. Too much bigness, too much wonderment – too much responsibility. For if you are God's equal, that means nothing is being done to you – and all things are created by you.

> There can be no more victims and no more
> villains – only outcomes of your thought
> about a thing.
>   I tell you this: all you see in your
> world is the outcome of your idea about it.
>   Do you want your life to truly "take
> off?" Then change your idea about it. About
> you. Think, speak, and act as the God you
> are."

Think about it. What does it mean to know that you
are the vibration of God? For one, if God has no limits,
then we have no limits. We say that God can heal. In fact
what can God not do? We also say that God is love,
which means that this is what we are too if we are one
with God. Is it surprising at all, then, that love heals? Or
that we can heal ourselves by aligning ourselves with our
true essence? This is a major premise of spiritual
traditions. Interestingly, it is also a major premise of the
science of quantum physics.

Quantum Physics

Lynn McTaggart has written an excellent book
tilted, *The Field: The Quest for the Secret Force of the
Universe,* which led her to understand scientifically the
meaning of interconnection and oneness. She reviewed
considerable research and interviewed many scientists,
especially physicists. She says:

> What they have discovered is nothing
> less than astonishing. At our most
> elemental, we are not a chemical reaction,
> but an energetic charge. Human Beings and

all living things are a coalescence of energy in a field of energy connected to every other thing in the world. This pulsating energy field is the central engine of our being and our consciousness, the alpha and the omega of our existence.

There is no 'me' and 'not-me' duality to our bodies in relation to the universe, but one underlying energy field. This field is responsible for our mind's highest functions, the information source guiding the growth of our bodies. It is our brain, our heart, our memory – indeed, a blueprint of the world for all time. The field is the force, rather than germs or genes, that finally determines whether we are healthy or ill, the force which must be tapped in order to heal. We are attached and engaged, indivisible from our world, and our only fundamental truth is our relationship with it. 'The field,' as Einstein once succinctly put it, 'is the only reality.'

Quantum physics is the study of electromagnetic energy at the atomic level. Its discovery about 100 years ago has raised radical questions scientifically about the nature of reality. Physicist Max Planck is considered the founder of quantum theory, and received a Nobel Prize in Physics in 1918, based on his discovery that a more fundamental quantum energy underlies all physical matter, and that so-called empty space is teeming with this energy. Einstein's theory of relativity concluded that space and time are not "fixed", and that the universe is constantly expanding. Along with other major physicists, including Erwin Schrödinger, Werner Heisenberg, and Niels Bohr, eventually it was determined that the universe was a dynamic web of interconnection.

Entanglement and Nonlocality

Neils Bohr received the Nobel Prize in Physics in 1922. Among his many discoveries, he determined that a tiny bundle of light energy called "quantum" emits photons (electromagnetic radiation), which became a basis for quantum theory. His principle of "complementarity" suggested that matter could behave either as a wave or particle. Werner Heisenberg was awarded the Nobel Prize in Physics in 1932 for his "uncertainty" principle that stated that it is not possible to know exactly both a definite position and a definite momentum of an electron. In 1933 Erwin Schrödinger was granted the Nobel Prize in Physics for his mathematical "equation" describing electrons in terms of waves as an alternative to the quantum theory of Heisenberg. All of them believed that the act of observation changes the phenomenon being observed. Reality as we think of it doesn't exist until we observe or measure it. There is no "fixed" reality. The quantum world is one of infinite potential that doesn't take form until consciousness is introduced.

However, when Einstein published his theory of relativity in 1915, a major premise was that any interaction between two separate particles could not take place faster than the speed of light. However, by 1935 quantum physicists were proposing that separated particles had the ability to communicate, or affect each other, instantaneously. Einstein then published what has become the most cited of his papers, attempting to reconcile these apparent anomalies. He wrote that there were "hidden variables" that could explain this – what he called "spooky action at a distance." The idea that something could not be objectively measured, or travel faster than the speed of light, did not suit his scientific theory. He could not accept theories of physics suggesting a universe of probabilities vs. certainties; thus his famous quote, "God does not play dice." Erwin Schrödinger was the first to publish a paper discussing Einstein's "spooky action at a distance" theory using the term "entangled" to explain this extraordinary phenomenon. In fact, he called this entangled quantum state "the characteristic trait of quantum physics".

Physics, like all science, is based on objective measurement. Galileo and Isaac Newton were two of the first great physicists to demonstrate that a theory must be strongly supported by controlled observations. Their observations confirmed what is now called the "mechanics" of the laws of motion and related forces, such as gravity. When Neils Bohr and others proposed that atomic and subatomic matter are ultimately "indeterminate" (that electron trajectories cannot be measured), Einstein rightly argued that any "element of physical reality" that could not be measured with certainty should not be included in quantum mechanics theory.

Physical reality to Einstein meant that "entangled" pairs of particles couldn't interact faster than the speed of light, as I've already noted. This is called a "local" effect. Therefore, any quantum mechanics theory that allowed for the non-separability of quantum particles did not measure up to this "locality assumption" or "local realism." Thus, we have the terms "entangled" or "quantum entanglement" and "local" or "locality" introduced to the scientific literature, which carry over today in the discussion of "nonlocality" and the interconnectedness of all of nature.

When physicist John Bell demonstrated conclusively in 1964 that information could be exchanged between two particles faster than the speed of light, he became the one most recognized at that time for discovering that nature is nonlocal and interconnected. His research was instrumental in establishing the science of quantum theory, and that there is an invisible force or energy, which unites all matter. The outcome of his research is commonly known as Bell's theorem, which essentially says that no physical theory of local hidden variables can ever explain or reproduce all of the predictions of quantum mechanics.

Many significant studies have since offered proof of Bell's theorem and nonlocal conclusion. There is now compelling evidence that quantum entanglement takes place both at the atomic and subatomic levels. One study in particular puts an exclamation point on the research supporting the oneness or connectedness of everything.

In 1997, physicist Nicholas Gisin and his colleagues at the University of Geneva clearly demonstrated a quantum connection in a rather spectacular experiment. They split a proton in two, and sent the pair of protons in opposite directions along optical fibers so that they were seven miles apart. The photons were then forced to choose between alternate random pathways. Even though they were separated miles apart, they always chose the exact same pathway. Whatever stimulus was applied to one of the protons, the other responded identically *instantaneously*.

Classical physics approaches continue to wrestle with the whys and hows of quantum entanglement. However, this evidence has given decided credibility, and spurred further research into Max Planck's original discovery of quantum and how these particles behave. In 1944, three years before his death, in his speech on "The Nature of Matter," Planck delivered his famous quote:

> As a man who has devoted his whole life to the most clear headed science, to the study of matter, I can tell you as a result of my research about atoms this much: There is no matter as such. All matter originates and exists only by virtue of a force which brings the particle of an atom to vibration and holds this most minute solar system of the atom together. We must assume behind this force the existence of a conscious and intelligent mind. This mind is the matrix of all matter.

Primary Perception

Cleve Backster's research always has stood out for me as another excellent demonstration of a quantum field effect and oneness. He is best known for his work with lie detectors and the fact that plants can sense human thought. Back in the 1960's he was curious if the lie detector (polygraph galvanic skin response or GSR) could measure how long it took for water to travel from the roots of a plant to its leaves. He assumed that the watering of the plant would register as a decreased electrical resistance response as the water reached a leaf of the plant where he had placed electrodes. But he got the opposite response. Curiously, the polygraph reading was typical of a human's reaction to emotional stimulation. After some thought, and as odd as it seemed at the time, it occurred to him that the plant was possibly demonstrating a human-like emotional reaction. Was it possible that the plant could have a similar sentient response?

So, he decided to "threaten" the plant by placing one of the plant's leaves in a hot cup of coffee. When the plant did not react, he decided that he needed a greater threat, and thought to get a match and burn the leaf. What he observed was a dramatic reaction on the GSR at the very moment of his thought. He didn't burn the leaf; he only thought to do it. The plant could read his mind!

Backster went on to research extensively, in controlled laboratory experiments, that plants were very sensitive to their environment and other living things. Plants reacted to threats to other plants and even bacteria. He proposed that there must be what he called a primary perception in plants.

Of special note was his research with human cells. He found that leukocytes taken from a lab volunteer named Steve White reacted wildly when Steve was looking through *Playboy* magazine to find a particular interview article, and saw Bo Derek "in her nothingness".

> ...His [White's] *in vitro* white cells showed full scale reaction hitting the top and bottom limit stops on the chart recorder.
> After two full minutes of continuous reactivity, I [Backster] suggested that he

close the magazine. When Steve closed the magazine his electroded cells calmed down as he attempted a process of mental disassociation. Then, a minute later, when he reached over to again open the closed magazine, the cells spiked again... it was the end of any raw skepticism about our research.

Later controlled research demonstrated primary perception, or what he called human cell "bio-communication", over distances of 50 miles. Interestingly, he found that intense emotions, such as whenever people felt threatened, registered more strongly than "loving and kind interactions". Backster first published this human cell research in the *International Journal of Biosocial Research* in 1985.

Later, Col. John Alexander, who was Chief of Advanced Human Technology at the U.S. Army Intelligence and Security Command, asked Backster to replicate his human cell research at their agency's headquarters. Backster describes two of the twelve studies in his book, *Primary Perception*. In each study people had leukocytes taken from the mouth in a saline solution so that they could be monitored for any reaction to their experiencing various emotions while watching television. The people were separated anywhere from ten blocks to fifteen miles from their donated white cells. When they experienced life threatening scenes, sexual imagery, emotionally charged family situations, or rage, their electroded cells registered dramatic reactions at the moment of their emotional experience while watching TV.

In later research with the army, DNA was taken from inside of a volunteer's mouth with a swab of tissue. As before, the donor viewed a series of emotionally charged images on TV. Although he was hundreds of feet away from his DNA, the DNA reacted dramatically again at the exact instant that the donor experienced various emotions.

Gregg Braden discusses this research in his book, *The Divine Matrix*. He talked with Backster personally about these studies. Backster confided that following the Army experiments, he did additional research where the donor was separated 350 miles from his cells. They had the same results. There was no time lapse between the cells' reaction and the person's emotions. Braden noted that the experiment suggests four things:

1. A previously unrecognized form of energy exists between living tissues.
2. Cells and DNA communicate through this field of energy.
3. Human emotion has a direct influence on living DNA.
4. Distance appears to be of no consequence with regard to the effect.

Braden then asks a highly relevant question, "How can the DNA react as if it were still connected to the donor's body in some way?" He proposed that:

If there's a quantum field that links all matter, then everything must be – and remain – connected. As Dr. Jeffrey Thompson, a colleague of Cleve Backster, states so eloquently, from this viewpoint: "There is no place where one's body actually ends and no place where it begins."

Dr. Myra Crawford, who is on faculty at the University of Alabama School of Medicine, visited Backster's lab in 2002 to look at his research. She had her own leukocytes extracted, and observed them react to her own emotional changes. She later wrote that she was indebted to Backter's research and its implications: "I have been shown in a scientific demonstration, the reality of conscious, non-local, instantaneous communication between my thoughts and my cells."

This research was later replicated with blood drawn from Dr. Crawford's assistant at the Institute of HeartMath's laboratory. After 36 years of research Backster believes that the mechanism of primary perception and the related bio-communication phenomena are best explained by current concepts within quantum physics, including that nonlocality consciousness pervades all of life.

Because human cells can be affected by thoughts and emotions, he concludes that illness could result from the expression or suppression of negative thoughts or emotions. "Additional study might more realistically reinforce reasons for positive thinking and for more effective management of one's emotions."

For those of you who are interested in pursuing more information and evidence of nonlocality, nonlocal mind, and how these might be applied in healing, I strongly recommend the physician and author, Dr. Larry Dossey. He is one of the true pioneers of mind-body-spirit medicine. Beginning with his book, *Space, Time, and*

Medicine, and every book since, he has a wonderful way of gathering great amounts of information and presenting it in a very meaningful and understandable way. The premise in his 1999 book, *Reinventing Medicine*, is that the mind is infinite, and that all minds are linked together. The mind is not localized or confined to the body, and healing is based on the fundamental infinite nature of consciousness.

Now I'd like to tell you briefly about primary perception in animals, but you probably already know this because of your own experience with your pets. Your pets positively can read your mind. Rupert Sheldrake asks in his book, *Dogs That Know When Their Owners Are Coming Home*, "How do cats and dogs and horses know when it's time to go to the vet, or go for a walk, or find their way home?" After many years of research with thousands of animals, pet owners, veterinarians, and animal trainers, he has found conclusively that animals have a sense of telepathy or "knowing" that can't be explained by behavioral cues or routines, or other conditioning. He believes that this bond with humans is related to "morphogenic fields" and a resonance that links animal-to-animal, person-to-person, and a person to a pet animal. There is an energetic connectedness among all of life. I'll say much more about this in the next chapter.

My friend Ken McCaulley discovered this connection with animals through his fascination with parapsychology. He said he met a lot of "kooks" in the process, but I remember one story in particular that got both of our attentions. When people heard that Ken was investigating psychic phenomena, they would sometimes plead with him to show him what often amounted to pet tricks, which were clearly learned and not paranormal.

One woman said that she could communicate mentally with her dog, and that it would do pretty much whatever she said.

She told Ken to whisper in her ear what he would like the dog to do. This was very unusual in Ken's experience. If he told her what to tell the dog, then this was not just some planned trick she taught her dog. So, Ken whispered to tell the dog to get up from where it was sleeping, and go over to a particular table, walk around it three times, then lay down again. What are the odds that she could get the dog to do this by simply asking it mentally? I don't think many of you, including Ken, believed she could do it, except she did!

Ken shared with me lots of unusual experiences like this. Another one that I remember well had to do with his garden. He had to go out of town for an extended time, and he was concerned about weeds growing, and animals getting into the yard and eating his plants and flowers. So, he mentally told the weeds to stop growing, and erected a "mental" fence to protect his garden. When he returned home, his garden was untouched and weed-free!

Years later I had an opportunity to demonstrate this for myself. My wife and I lived on a twelve-acre property that was surrounded by much larger neighboring properties. There was lots of wildlife that lived and wandered through our land. Plus we had a 1-½ acre pond that attracted them even more. So, when we wanted to build a ¼ acre garden, I was very concerned that it would be eaten by the gophers, deer, turkeys, and geese, in particular. We built a seven-foot fence, but how do you keep the moles, voles, gophers, and birds out?

So, I talked to them. Every day for months I told the wildlife that they were welcome on our property, but they had to stay outside of the garden fence. Fat chance, huh? Except it worked. It almost worked too well. Seemingly every gopher-like creature in the world showed up on our property. But they didn't burrow under into the garden! I figured that if we were all one, and connected somehow, it was worth a try. And it worked. Thank you, "infinite mind."

The Right Brain Hemisphere

A recent example of oneness can be found in the fascinating 2008 book, *My Stroke of Insight*, by Dr. Jill Bolte Taylor. It is a perfect blend of science, personal experience, and insight. It is a *New York Times* bestseller, and her 18-minute video on TED.com has become an Internet favorite. *Time* magazine chose her as one of the "Most Influential People in the World for 2008".

Jill is a neuroanatomist and on faculty at the Indiana School of Medicine. In 1996 she had a stroke, and because of her being a brain scientist, she understood exactly what was happening to her. She claims to have learned as much about the function of the brain from her personal experience of the stroke as from all of her study and training. Her insights into the unique functions of the right and left hemispheres of the brain were startling.

Jill explains how the left hemisphere works to categorize, organize, describe, judge and critically analyze everything we perceive. It is a master multi-tasker and loves theorizing, rationalizing, and memorizing. It is a do-er and mental obsessor, unlike the right hemisphere, which lives in the moment and thrives on being the "nonjudgmental witness." Both hemispheres work together to determine our truth and reality. But their truths are very different.

The left hemisphere's truth is remarkably subjective, based on learned and conditioned beliefs and perceptions. This is where the ego resides. Its job is to help us survive in the world. It views itself as individual, solid, separate, and limited by physical boundaries.

However, Jill found quite by surprise that the right hemisphere knows a very different reality. Because the left half of her brain was impaired by her stroke, she lost the ability to organize and analyze information. She found the absence of the perception of physical boundaries to be "one of glorious bliss". She knew, as the brain scientist, that everything was energy, "spinning and vibrating atomic particles." We live in and are part of a "sea of electromagnetic fields". And now she was experiencing a consciousness that was a "silent euphoria" and "a flow of sweet tranquility." She was no longer bound to her prior learned beliefs about who she was. She now learned the meaning of simply "being". Released from the restrictive circuitry of her left hemisphere, she found herself in an "eternal flow". Her "soul was as big as the universe, and frolicked with glee in a boundless sea".

Jill acknowledges that thinking about ourselves this way is out of the "comfort zone" for many of us. But without the use of left-brain judgment, she found herself in a "natural state of fluidity". The energy of electrons, protons, and neutrons that make up the physical world were no longer perceived as separate from one another. Everything blended together and was "connected to the energy flow of all that is". All flowed together as *one*.

It was "an unforgettable sense of peace". She found we are connected to, and a part of all that is. There was no fear. Our perception of the physical universe is a product of our left hemisphere circuitry. Her right hemisphere knew her as "simply a being of light radiating life into the world...", "a cellular masterpiece...", and "perfect, whole, and beautiful just the way I was." Her consciousness now was one of "eternal bliss" and "deep inner peace". This became her stroke of insight, which is the premise of her book: *peace is only a thought away, and all we have to do to access it is silence the voice of our dominating left mind*.

True bliss, peace and calm are available to anyone at any time. This is our natural state. Unlike the left hemisphere that is concerned with pleasing others, and seeking their approval, the right hemisphere "is completely committed to the expression of peace, love, joy, and compassion in the world". Neuroanatomy research had already discovered that certain regions of the brain became more active during meditative spiritual or mystical experiences. She now was living this shift in consciousness – "away from being an individual to feeling that we are at *one* with the universe (God, Nirvana, euphoria)". She notes that the left brain is doing the best it can with the information it has been given, but we can consciously choose to realign with the present moment, and become free of negative thoughts and fears.

Jill reports that these normal fears and emotions take about 90 seconds to run their course as a natural physiological response. Her advice is to pay attention to our self-talk, and to honor any negative thoughts or emotions. But once they've run their 90-second course, then we need to instruct our left brain that this negative focus is no longer acceptable. You'll remember that your left hemisphere genuinely wants you to be happy and healthy. It's just that it has faulty information to work with. It needs to be retrained. You have to change and break former beliefs and associations.

For example, in the psychological principle of "reciprocal inhibition", you inhibit one response by pairing it with a response with which it is mutually incompatible. For example, if you were anxious, but immediately thought or did something that was relaxing, eventually whatever was creating the anxiety would dissipate. You can't be anxious and relaxed at the same time. This approach is used in what is called "desensitization", and is one of the most researched and effective of all behavior therapies.

Thus, Jill recommends that whenever you feel out of sorts, wait 90 seconds, then focus on something positive like your pet animal, grandchild, favorite activity, or anything that has special meaning for you. It's hard to feel stressed if you're having fun. She also offers numbers of suggestions to slow down our minds, and bring us into the present moment. Then as we shift into our right mind, our intuitive wisdom kicks in and we perceive a bigger picture where "everything is woven together into a universal tapestry".

She says that if she had to define her right mind with one word, it would be *compassion*. And when we are being compassionate, we act with love and empathy, not judgment or fear or aggression. If she had to pick one word to describe the feeling at the core of her right brain, it would be *joy*; "happiness is the natural state of being for my right mind". When she remembers that she is *one* with the universe, "the concept of fear loses its power".

Jill believes that her stroke was the best thing that ever happened to her. She learned that you could shift your perception from your logical left brain hemisphere to the right intuitive hemisphere, and experience a completely different reality of peace and well-being. She now encourages meditation and yoga as a way to balance the brain, where we can capitalize on the unique gifts of both hemispheres. A sense of feeling at one with the universe is our true and natural state. Mystical or metaphysical experiences have a basis in fact. She has come to a very different understanding of mind, emotions, energy, healing, and reality.

Chapter 5 - Mind, Emotions, and Energy

In Chapters 1 and 2 I briefly introduced that I had studied guided imagery as part of my doctoral dissertation, and that I taught guided imagery as part of my program for cancer patients. I had learned about it first in 1977 from Ken McCaulley, and used it personally to realize the remarkable ability of the mind to heal. Indeed, after more than 30 years of practice and study, I can attest clinically and scientifically to the effectiveness of mind-body approaches in general. When Dr. Martin Rossman and I co-authored a chapter on "Mind-Body Medicine in Integrative Cancer Care" in the book, *Integrative Oncology* (2009), we were surprised to find just how much research now exists supporting the use of guided imagery with cancer. Rather than attempt to cite all of the studies in our chapter, we opted to cite just some of the meta-analyses, because there were so many, all of which reported positive outcomes.

Most commonly, guided imagery is explained as a result of the placebo effect, or what you might understand as "sugar pills." It's based on your beliefs or expectations. If a physician prescribed a medication, and you took it, you generally would expect to get well. Assuming that you believe in the expertise of your doctor, and if your doctor told you to take this medication, you probably would take it and would feel better. However, if your doctor gave you a placebo or "sugar pills" (fake pills, pills with no active substance in them), but you didn't know they were fake, you would still get better about one-third of the time. If we don't control for the placebo effect in conducting research, the research in fact has no merit scientifically. That's how important and powerful your beliefs are.

This is why drugs are tested and compared to a placebo because your *belief* that you are getting treatment can bring about the same results as the actual treatment. This is why we have "double-blind" studies. Here, neither the physician (nor anyone administering the treatment) nor the patient knows which is the real treatment or medication. This is because not only can the patients' beliefs affect the outcome, so can the doctors'. This is an excellent scientific demonstration of the power of your mind.

When I wrote my doctoral dissertation, I surveyed the scientific literature and actually found there were ten hypotheses that explained the effectiveness of guided imagery. (These can be found in *Doctor's Orders: Go Fishing*). The tenth hypothesis states, "Guided imagery is consistent with holographic theory, quantum mechanics, and theoretical physics." I cited physicist David Bohm in particular, who believed that there is an infinite sea of energy that underlies and unfolds to form space, time, and matter. All of reality is a manifestation of this deeper energy, a matrix of harmony and order. Underlying all of these energy patterns or vibratory fields of energy is a "Primary Reality," which is the source of all other realities.

Implicit in this theory is that harmonious states of consciousness are more attuned to this primary, underlying reality. Attunement, then, would be difficult in states of anxiety and stress, and be facilitated by states such as relaxation and meditation. When you are in a deep state of relaxation as part of practicing guided imagery, any thoughts and feelings, while in a state of harmony, resonate with the underlying energy matrix of harmony and order (Primary Reality). And, thus, they could become manifest in reality. Therefore, your thoughts and prayers could actually create reality, or the visualization (guided imagery) could act as a guiding form or pattern for the energy to materialize.

Early quantum physicists, Bohr, Heisenberg, and Schrödinger's research concluded that subatomic matter is really interacting waves of "potential" energy that only takes physical form once observed. An electron only takes shape and can be measured once it is actually being measured. The observation of a thing takes it from its undefined waveform of pure potential and only then does it appear as a particle or atomic matter. Consciousness is necessary for the creation of matter and the physical universe! This again suggests that your mind, and the specific application of your mind in the use of guided imagery or prayer, could literally create a specific outcome.

Dr. Richard Conn Henry is a Professor of Physics and Astronomy at Johns Hopkins University. His article titled, "The Mental Universe" published in 2005 in the prestigious science journal, *Nature*, states, "The only reality is mind and observations, but observations are not things. To see the Universe as it really is, we must abandon our tendency to conceptualize observations as things." He cited physicist Sir James Jeans, who said, "...the Universe begins to look more like a great thought than like a great machine. Mind no longer appears to be an accidental intruder into the realm of matter." Henry noted that historically, religions have been the ones to give understanding to the nature of our world, but that physics has "joined religion in seeking to explain our place in the Universe." He concluded his article, "The Universe is immaterial – mental and spiritual."

Another eminent Princeton physicist, John Wheeler, who was a colleague of Einstein's, calls this a "participatory universe." Our observations, expectations, and beliefs literally create our world. We're the intelligent mind that Planck proposed underlies the creation of the universe.

The Law of Attraction

An often-cited quote of the Buddha is, "If you want peace, be peace." Or, as Gandhi said, "Be the change you want to see in the world." You need to be aligned with what you want. This is related to the idea that you reap what you sow. Remember: Consciousness creates. Whatever you put your attention on, you create or attract.

Esther and Jerry Hicks have written about this extensively in their many books. My favorite is *Ask and It is Given*, written in 2004. Many of you may be familiar with these books, including one titled *The Law of Attraction*, written in 2006. The basic premise of these books is that you are the creator of your experience. You create your own reality. Many of you also may be familiar with the DVD and book, *The Secret*. This information is based largely on the teachings of Esther and Jerry Hicks.

When I read *Ask and It is Given* the first time, and especially the processes and exercises that were recommended in the book, I wasn't fully ready to accept and apply them. I was dealing with my own control issues and a certain amount of dissatisfaction with where I was in my life. When I reread it a year or so later, I knew instantly that I not only wanted to apply this information, I needed to teach it. I immediately called my office and scheduled a date to teach a class on "The Law of Attraction: Why 'The Secret' Works, and Why It Doesn't." It became very important for me to explain how this law of attraction works to help people get what they really want out of life. And I also wanted to respond to people who were claiming that "The Secret" doesn't work.

The DVD and the book titled "The Secret" became very popular in 2007. It was given extensive coverage on major programs such as Oprah and the Larry King Show. And like anything, it had its detractors. Articles appeared saying that it was too simplistic and that it didn't really work. I knew that it worked, and I needed and wanted to explain why and how. Actually, the law of attraction made great sense to me all along. It correlated well with my study and practice of guided imagery and now with my study of quantum physics. In an article from her website, "The Secret Behind 'The Secret'," Lynn McTaggart explains:

> At the nethermost level of reality – the realm of the quantum particle – we are not separate 'things' but vibrating energy connected by a vast quantum energy field. Subatomic particles resemble little packets of vibrating waves, passing energy back and forth as if in an endless game of basketball. These back-and-forth passes, which rise to an extraordinarily large ground state of energy, are known collectively as the Zero

Point Field. The very underpinning of our universe is this heaving sea of energy – one vast quantum field, with everything held in its invisible web. On our most fundamental level, living beings are packets of quantum energy constantly exchanging information with this inexhaustible energy sea...

The only thing dissolving this little cloud of potential into something solid and measurable is the involvement of an observer. Once these scientists have a closer look at a subatomic particle by taking a measurement, the subatomic entity that existed as pure potential 'collapses' into one particular state.

The implications of quantum experimental findings are profound: The moment we look at an electron or take a measurement, *it appears that we help to determine its final state*. This suggests that the most essential ingredient in creating our universe is the consciousness that observes it.

The Hicks are clear in *Ask and It Is Given* regarding the law of attraction, saying that it is helpful to think of ourselves as a "Vibrational Being" because everything in the universe is energy or vibration. And every thought we have is an energy that radiates a signal and attracts a matching signal back. Like attracts like. You reap what you sow. Whatever you think about the most becomes a practiced or dominant thought, and *"Once your focused attention has sufficiently activated a dominant vibration* *within you, <u>things</u> – wanted and unwanted – will begin to make their way into your personal experience. It is law."*

This means that it's important to focus on what you want vs. what you don't want. This is the greatest reason why the law of attraction or "The Secret" doesn't work: People don't realize that every thought and feeling affects what they attract into their life experience. They don't understand that they are often spending considerable time worrying and thinking about what they don't want. Similarly, you can't focus on a desire and expect it to happen if it's more like a "yearning", and a significant focus is your awareness of its absence. Worry is insidiously unproductive and unhealthy. Consider even the examples of well-meaning, but counter productive intentions such as: Say "no" to drugs vs. Say "yes" to healthy lifestyles, "War is not the answer" vs. "Give peace a chance," and a Department of War vs. a Department of Peace. The Hicks state:

> Often – even when you believe you are thinking about something that you desire – you are actually thinking about the exact opposite of what you desire. In other words, "I want to be well; I don't want to be sick." "I want to have financial security; I don't want to experience a shortage of money." "I want the perfect relationship to come to me; I don't want to be alone."
> *What you think and what you get is always a perfect vibrational match...*

The very good news is that you and "Source" (the term that the Hicks prefer when referring to God) are the same vibration. You can hinder your connection with Source when your thoughts are different enough in vibrational nature from Source, but you can never be separate from your Divine Nature or True Self. Resistant thoughts such as impatience, doubt, pessimism, worry, discouragement, anger, insecurity, depression and unworthiness are the only things stopping you from getting what you want. There is only a flow of "Well-Being" or Source Energy. You can allow it or resist it.

What is key here are any thoughts or feelings of separation from Divine Source. This forms a disconnect with who you truly are. It creates a dissonance, and disrupts the flow of "Well-Being," life force energy, or connection with the quantum field. Your connection with Source can only bring well-being. As the Hicks say in *Ask and It Is Given*, "there is no dark switch; there is no Source of 'evil' or Source of sickness or lack."

> *All the resources you will ever want or need are at your fingertips. All you have to do is identify what you want to do with it and then practice the feeling-place of what it will be like when that happens.* There is nothing you cannot be, do, or have; you are blessed Beings, and you have come forth into this physical environment to create. There is nothing holding you back other than your own contradictory thoughts.

Not only do your thoughts create reality, your very purpose for being in human form is to experience the joy and thrill of creation. You are Eternal Consciousness, Divine Vibration – the very same vibration as God or

Source Energy. You are a co-creator with God. "The basis of life is freedom… but the purpose of your life is joy." Discomfort or any negative feeling is feedback that you are resisting the flow of Source Energy.

This is why I'm so grateful for my training and experience in guided imagery, relaxation, meditation, and mind-body medicine. We need to relax. Whenever we find ourselves focusing on what we don't want, or feeling out-of-sorts, we need to refocus on something positive – gently. Or go fishing. Do what brings you joy, a zest for life, a will to live. The Hicks believe that there is no better guidance than to follow your bliss, for then "you must surely align with the Energy of your Source." This is the secret. Find your joy, and you have found the secret.

Quantum theory and research tell us that this is a participatory universe. Our thoughts create. Matter only becomes a physical reality through the focus of our attention. Whatever we're thinking and feeling literally causes that very thing to take form. And metaphysics informs us similarly of the law of attraction. You create your own reality. Consciousness is the key.

Morphogenetic and Life Fields

Biochemist Dr. Rupert Sheldrake calls this focused consciousness "formative causation." Thought gives form to something in the same way that an architectural blueprint gives form to a building. The thought or blueprint creates the energy field that determines the form. This energy field attracts suitable energetic material or "building blocks," which become the physical structure. Sheldrake calls these field-structures "morphogenetic fields." The more these thought-forms or fields are repeated increases the probability of that physical outcome.

I first read about this in his book, *A New Science of Life: The Hypothesis of Formative Causation* when I was in graduate school. It fascinated me so much that I read the whole book in one night. This sure gave credence and a way to understand the effectiveness of guided imagery. In his book *The Presence of the Past: Morphic Resonance and the Habits of Nature*, he agrees with Sir Arthur Eddington that "the stuff of the world is mind stuff".

While I was reviewing the scientific literature regarding guided imagery I also discovered the research of Dr. Harold Saxton Burr. Burr was E.K. Hunt Professor of Anatomy at Yale University School of Medicine. I read numbers of his journal articles and his books, *The Fields of Life: Our Links With the Universe* and *The Nature of Man and The Meaning of Existence*. His research concluded that there was an electromagnetic field that functioned as a blueprint-like mold for all living organisms. He was able to measure this "L-field", which stands for fields of life, in humans, animals, trees, plants, seeds, eggs, and even slime-molds. He offered this example in *The Fields of Life* to explain how these electromagnetic fields organize and maintain life:

> ...If iron filings are scattered on a card held over a magnet they will arrange themselves in the pattern of the 'lines of force' of the magnet's field. And if the filings are thrown away and fresh ones scattered on the card, the new filings will assume the same pattern as the old.

Something like this – though infinitely more complicated – happens in the human body. Its molecules and cells are constantly being torn apart and rebuilt with fresh material from the food we eat. But, thanks to the controlling L-field, the new molecules are rebuilt as before and arrange themselves in the same pattern as the old ones.

There is an energy matrix, a primary electrodynamic field that shapes the living form.

Burr further found that one's state of mind is reflected in the state of the field. Worries could produce illness. Emotions have a definite reality. He noted that, "an idea is just as valid a stimulus to the nervous system as a kick in the teeth."

These electrodynamic fields direct the chemical, metabolic and molecular transformations of an organism. Additional research by Dr. Leonard Ravitz confirmed that these fields "serve basic functions, controlling growth and morphogenesis, maintenance and repair of living things…serving as an electronic matrix to keep the corporal form in shape." His later research showed that this L-field disappears before physical death.

Psychoneuroimmunology

In Chapter 2, I mentioned research in psychoneuroimmunology, the study of how your emotional state interacts with your immune system. Prior to the 1970's it was believed that one's thoughts or feelings couldn't affect the disease process because the central nervous system and the immune system were not linked. Think about it. If your immune system functioned independently of every other system, meaning that your brain and spinal cord (central nervous system) were not connected to your immune system, how could your emotional state contribute to disease? Forget the common sense notion that if you're feeling happy or sad, relaxed or tense, that this would affect your health. Until now there was no known biological or biochemical mechanism for this to be able to happen. But in the 1970's this new field of study, psychoneuroimmunology, emerged that would radically change the notion of mind and body being separate.

Dr. Robert Ader, a psychologist at the University of Rochester School of Medicine, and a colleague, Dr. Nicholas Cohen, an immunologist, found that if you paired a drug which suppresses immune function with a placebo, eventually the immune system becomes suppressed by the placebo alone. This is similar to Pavlov's pairing the ringing of a bell with presenting meat to a dog. Eventually the ringing of the bell alone, without the meat, caused the dog to salivate because of the association of the bell with food. He called this "classical conditioning," a form of learning. Learning does not take place without the use of a brain. In order for the placebo in Ader and Cohen's research to suppress immune function through this form of learning, the brain had to be connected to the immune system. Further research demonstrated that this same "conditioning" approach could enhance immune function and decrease the side effects of toxic chemotherapeutic drugs, such as those used to treat cancer.

Dr. Ader coined the term "psychoneuro-immunology" to account for the interaction between learning (psycho), implicating the physical brain (neuro), and one's immune function. He edited the now-classic text called *Psychoneuroimmunology* in 1981. Each chapter is original research clearly demonstrating a link between the central nervous system and the immune system. This confirmed the earlier research of Dr. George Solomon who coined the term "psychoimmunology" to explain how personality affects disease.

Much research has been done since to confirm that the immune system is capable of self-regulation. In 1985, *The Journal of Immunology* devoted a special issue just to research demonstrating the interaction of the central nervous and immune system. A principal investigator in one of these studies was Dr. Candace Pert, who was then Chief of Brain Biochemistry for the National Institutes of Mental Health. Her research demonstrated that the immune system is in constant communication with the brain, endocrine and nervous systems by a system of peptides. In her book, *Molecules of Emotion*, Pert says that she prefers to call these peptides "informational substances – because it points to their common function, that of messenger molecules distributing information throughout the organism". These peptide structures previously have been classified under a wide variety of categories, including hormones, transmitters, neurotransmitters, neuromodulators, growth factors, gut peptides, interleukins, cytokines, chemokines, and growth-inhibiting factors.

In her books, *Molecules of Emotion* and *Everything You Need to Know to Feel Go(o)d*, she explains how emotions are actually physical substances (receptors and peptides) that convey information throughout the body. She details a psychosomatic network that explains the biochemical basis of how emotions affect health or disease. Through simple biochemistry she describes how the body and mind are actually one, which she calls the "bodymind".

Virtually every cell in the body has thousands of receptors. Signals from other cells come from hormones, neurotransmitters, and peptides. Usually these are all referred to as ligands, which means, "to bind," because of the way they attract and bind to cell receptors. This used to be thought of as a lock and key relationship, where a peptide (key) would insert itself into a receptor (lock) to affect cellular activity. It is now known that there also is a vibratory attraction between ligands vibrating at the same frequency. This cellular resonance is the emotion, and the actual connection, (peptide to receptor), manifests as feeling. That's why Pert calls peptides and their receptors the molecules of emotion.

This is not a cause-and-effect relationship. It's all happening simultaneously. As Pert explains in the following quotations from *Everything You Need to Know to Feel Go(o)d*:

> Molecules *are* the emotions, not their cause. What we experience as "feeling" is the actual vibrational dance that goes on when peptides bind to their receptors, whether it happens in your conscious awareness or not… This is why I say: *Your body is your subconscious mind.*

Pert notes that many ancient civilizations believed that consciousness is real and creates physical reality. Conventional science has it in reverse and believes that consciousness is a by-product of the physical. However, quantum physics theory and Pert believe that consciousness is in the body, as she explains:

> But contrary to the reigning-paradigm belief, the body doesn't exist merely to carry the head around! The body isn't an appendage dangling from the almighty brain that rules over all systems. Instead, the brain itself is one of many nodal, or entry, points into a dynamic network of communication that unites all systems – nervous, endocrine, immune, respiratory, and more. This is called the psychosomatic network, and the linking elements to keep it all together are the informational substances – peptides, hormones, and neurotransmitters – known as the molecules of emotion…
>
> Yes, your symptoms are in your body, but they are also *always* in your mind, either consciously or subconsciously. Mind and body are not split in two, so what happens in one occurs in the other, too. This is the fundamental tenet of what I call the new-paradigm physiology.

How you feel affects cell activity in much the same way as drugs. Pert believes that your attitude and emotions affect change in your body, including tumor progression or regression. Buried, painful emotions need to be gently brought to gradual awareness to be re-experienced, understood, and reintegrated. As we let go of old traumatic energy patterns, we become healed or whole. She concludes that if you want to feel good (and healthy), "Just love." Loving yourself and others "is our true spiritual heritage. When we're closely connected with each other, we're living as we were designed to do biologically, psychologically, and spiritually".

Pert contends that compassion is a quantum event, and that this caring is a resonant energy that can create a coherent, healing state. Feeling unconnected, alone, and not realizing that we're all one is the root of all fear. This is the underlying cause of not feeling good physically and emotionally.

Epigenetics

Another excellent example of the power of the mind and emotions comes from the research of cell biologist, Dr. Bruce Lipton, and a new field of study called epigenetics. Epigenetics is the study of non-genetic factors that cause an organism's genes to express or behave differently. Dr. Lipton has written an excellent article, "The Wisdom of Your Cells", explaining his research and epigenetics, which can be found on his website (www.brucelipton.com). Lipton began his training at the University of Wisconsin in the 1960's working with Dr. Irv Konigsberg, who created the first stem cell cultures. He quickly discovered that cells were controlled far more by their environment than their genetic makeup. When he put muscle cells in culture dishes with conditions that supported muscle growth, the muscles cells evolved into muscles. However, if he placed these same muscle cells in an altered environment, they would begin to form bone cells or fat cells depending on the cell environment, even though the cells were genetically identical!

He explains that every function of the body is inherently present in every cell. All of the functions of your bodily systems, including digestive, respiratory, excretory, musculoskeletal, endocrine, reproductive, nervous, and immune systems are in every one of your cells. His research revealed that the control center of the cell is its membrane or outer surface "skin". The cell membrane actually functions like an information-processing computer chip, and the cell's genes are the hard drive with all the potential to be any kind of cell. The genes respond (are turned on or off) by perceptions handled by the cell membrane.

In his book, *The Biology of Belief,* Lipton states that the conventional idea of genes controlling biology is a hypothesis, and is not proven. It is an assumption that the nucleus of a cell, and its DNA-containing material, control the cell. Laboratory research demonstrates that when you remove the cell's nucleus, the cell continues to survive for up to two or three months. If genes control the body, how does the cell continue to live without its genes? He says that eventually cells die because they have lost the ability to reproduce their parts (protein building blocks to replicate themselves).

More than one hundred thousand proteins act as receivers on the cell membrane and control the functions of our lives through awareness of the environment. These membrane "switches" perceive the environment and adjust our biology as a basic adaptation response. This was a major "aha" moment when he realized that "*perception controls behavior*". Rather than being the victim of our genes, or being biochemical machines – our thoughts, beliefs, and mind control our genes, our behavior, and the life we experience. We are very powerful creators, and determine the quality of our life and health. He notes that this is very hard for most people to accept.

There's a certain comfort in believing that all the signals that control our genes and biology are chemical. This is why pharmaceuticals were created. It was believed (and largely still is) that drugs or medication could manage regulation of the cell's proteins. However, to now have to accept personal responsibility for our thoughts and perceptions is both good news and bad news. The good news is that you are not powerless and that you can take control of your health and life. The bad news is that *you* have to do it.

Like Dr. Candace Pert, Lipton notes that our cells communicate far more through exchange of energy than chemically. Everything is made out of energy. Every atom in your body is constantly sending and receiving energy. Your body is a community of about 50 trillion living cells, and "health is when there is harmony in the community, and dis-ease is when there is a disharmony that tends to fracture the community relationships."

This concept of Lipton's explains why he believes that we need to live in harmony with nature. This is not a Darwinian "survival of the fittest." Evolution is based on cooperation. Everything is one whole. We are part of the quantum field, and our thoughts are part of this energy field.

Lipton found that any dysfunction or disease is a result of our proteins not having the right structure (genetic defects) or inappropriate environmental signals. However, he says that far less than five percent of the population has genetic defects. He goes on to say:

> That means ninety-five percent of us arrived on this planet with genes that were capable of providing us with a healthy existence. For ninety-five percent of the population, if they are failing in health it is not something wrong with the genes and proteins, it is something wrong with the body's *signals*. Inappropriate signals are the source of most human illnesses and dysfunctions.

He believes that the greatest source of incorrect signaling comes from the mind: perceived stress and fears. And when we are afraid, we naturally shift into the fight or flight response, which shuts down cell growth processes. Our cells are constantly engaged in either growth or protection mechanisms. They cannot do both at the same time. The more we live in fear and high levels of stress, our system begins to break down.

We are constantly losing and regenerating cells. And when we experience excessive stress, it can interfere with the ability to replace lost cells and also compromise bodily functions, including the immune system. This is why Lipton believes that almost every major illness is linked to chronic stress, including depression. At the extreme, as I explained in *Doctor's Orders: Go Fishing*: Stress can kill you.

Lipton explains in detail how our subconscious mind is the greatest source of life-controlling perceptions.

And this process begins in the womb. The mother's blood contains more than nutrients for the baby; it contains "information molecules" as well. Through the placenta, the baby experiences and is affected by the mother's emotional state. Mother's stress hormones register in the fetus.

Is the womb environment and energy field one of love and harmony? (Or as the Hicks would ask: Are you resonating with Source, and allowing Source or Life Force Energy to flow)? Parent's thoughts and feelings literally contribute to the child's physiology and behavior. Lipton states:

> If the parents find the world troubling, their child will be affected. For example, when parents do not want a child, this information, in the form of emotional chemistry, is crossing the placenta! The fetus already knows that its support is not guaranteed. It is clearly important for us to recognize that creating a child is a very important, dynamic, interactive process between the parents and the fetus. In fact, recent understanding in human pathology clearly reveals that issues that affect us as adults, such as cardiovascular disease, cancer and obesity, actually have their roots in the peri-conceptual, fetal and neonatal phases of life. The conditions under which a child is developing in utero profoundly shape her for the rest of her life in regard to behavior and physiology.

Our prenatal and childhood environments dramatically shape our beliefs about the world and ourselves, and have real consequences on our health. A fetus or infant doesn't have the use of reason or logic to rebut the beliefs of parents and other authority figures. It is like a sponge simply absorbing and responding to life around it. This creates the subconscious or egoic mind. It is a repository of our learned beliefs about who we are and what we need to do to survive. And what we learn to some extent (or a large extent) is that we're no good and unloved, and the only way to feel good about ourselves is when we're pleasing others. At a deep psychic level, we learn to equate conforming (pleasing others and adopting their beliefs) with being or feeling loved. (See *Doctor's Orders: Go Fishing*, Chapter 9 for an in-depth discussion of this process).

The good news is that you can change your beliefs, which sends totally different messages to your cells, and can reprogram their expression. In his website article, "Mind Over Genes: The New Biology", Lipton calls this new understanding the "new-biology". It incorporates the role of mind and spirit. "The new-biology reveals why people can have spontaneous remissions or recover from injuries deemed to be permanent disabilities."

He believes that our beliefs act like filters on a camera, changing how we see the world. And our biology adapts to those beliefs. We have come to believe that our genes, which control our biochemistry and health, have preprogrammed us. His research makes a convincing argument that by choosing different colored filters, we can take control of our life and change our health. Lipton states:

You can filter your life with rose-colored beliefs that will help your body grow or you can use a dark filter that turns everything black and makes your body/mind more susceptible to disease. You can live a life of fear or live a life of love. You have the choice! But I can tell you that if you choose to see a world full of love, your body will respond by growing in health. If you choose to believe that you live in a dark world full of fear, your body's health will be compromised as you physiologically close yourself down in a protection response.

Learning how to harness your mind to promote growth is the secret of life, which is why I called this book *The Biology of Belief*. Of course the secret of life is not a secret at all. Teachers like Buddha and Jesus have been telling us the same story for millennia. Now science is pointing in the same direction.

Chapter 6 - Empathy And Forgiveness

Even if you can grasp and accept that you are God–like, Divine Source Energy, love, and oneness, most people cannot or do not want to believe that in some way they have attracted everything and everyone in their life. The relationships and situations we find ourselves in are the mirror of our thoughts and feelings. It can actually function as a wonderful feedback system to let us see and learn about ourselves. It's also an excellent demonstration of our power to create. Your thoughts and feelings attract to you people and situations that directly reveal your deepest beliefs about yourself and the world. As Bruce Lipton just noted, we develop these beliefs early in life.

From day one we begin to react to our environment, doing our best to adapt and survive. We acquire beliefs from our parents, in particular, about what is right and wrong, who we are, and how we're supposed to present ourselves to the world. And when we violate any of these learned beliefs, we begin to develop guilt and shame. We develop a "shadow" side of our selves. We try to hide it and deny it, and one way to cope with these uncomfortable feelings is to suppress or repress them, and take them out of our conscious memory. Another way is to blame and project what we rejected or denied about ourselves onto others. In psychology this is called scape-goating or projection.

I'd really like you to think about this because if we could look at what we judge about ourselves and others, we could see it as a way to understand ourselves so much better. Truly, like the law of attraction, the people in your life (including your pets and co-workers) are mirrors of you – the good and the bad. It takes courage to accept that what we don't like about others is what we consciously or subconsciously don't want to acknowledge in ourselves.

Experiences of guilt, shame, and rejection are how your "inner critic" is born. Psychologists, Hal and Sidra Stone discuss this concept well in their book, *Embracing Your Inner Critic*. We all to some degree, early in life, develop insecurities and fears largely based on our parents' beliefs. And, like it or not, we become a lot like our parents. Actually, your inner critic is primarily the voice of your parents. As children, we may feel alone and afraid, and want to reach out for love and to feel safe, but we usually can't for fear of further rejection if we're not measuring up to our parents' or other's ideals.

In my case I developed my father's perfectionist tendencies, "If you're going to do something, do it right. You should be willing to sign your name to whatever you do." I similarly learned from him a definite defensiveness, rigidity, and cut off from my feelings: "If you want to cry, I'll give you something to cry about." I had to do it his way.

The research and common sense are that you feel best and are most healthy when you are able to be yourself, when you are being unique. You didn't learn to be unique. Most of us learned to conform to the beliefs and values of our parents. You weren't stupid – if you were going to be yelled at and made to feel unworthy and unloved for not obeying your parents or other authority figures, you're going to soon catch on. You learn to equate love with conforming.

Your inner critic, like your ego, is simply a survival mechanism doing its best to help you make it in the world. As you experience more and more thoughts and feelings of separation and fear vs. oneness and love, you subconsciously create aspects or sub personalities of yourself that you come to believe are who you really are. They include your inner critic, rule maker, pleaser, responsible parents, and other selves. These "selves" that you call your personality, were developed by your subconscious, and take over when you're feeling vulnerable. And your beliefs about who you are will be reflected in your primary relationships in particular. They are your mirrors.

In marriage, for example, you will attract someone who carries your "disowned selves", the parts you've somehow learned are socially unacceptable. I tend to say that you marry your opposite. One of the most common observations I've made is that one of you will be significantly more self-centered, and one of you will be more of a nurturer. One of you can't wait to throw things out, and the other wants to hoard and save. If you really think about this, it can make you wonder why in the world you married this person. You can be so different. The reason is that at an energetic level, you attract others to fill in your void and to balance you. Interestingly, all of the qualities that you are looking for in another are within you ("Oz never did give nothin' to the Tin Man that he didn't already have"). And those who push your buttons, or who you overvalue, are your best teachers. Your beliefs at a vibratory level attracted you to each other. If only we could see our relationships this way, and how we can help one another instead of judging and wanting to change them.

Interestingly, the best way to change them is to change yourself. As you learn to love and accept yourself, it changes your energy and the way others relate to you. If you change, they have to change also. Believe me, this doesn't always go smoothly, but the key is your becoming more aware of the truth of who you are and assuming a conscious, caring role in relation to "the inner critic". Your inner critic can become a special ability to spot problems, and a warning system that you're out of balance. This is the role of your emotions.

In their many books, Esther and Jerry Hicks refer to an "emotional guidance system." How you feel is an indication of how well you are aligned with the truth of who you are. Are you aligned with Divine Source, and allowing this Energy to flow? If so, you will feel good. This is the same with your health. A major premise in shamanism is that medical symptoms are what I call benevolent messengers. They're feedback letting you know that you're out of balance or alignment. And when you rebalance, your symptoms have no reason for being, and go away. If we are willing to be more introspective, and really see ourselves as a bunch of sub personalities that we have acquired, like our ego, as a misguided way to survive, we can begin to see our True Self. Ideally you want to meditate and really learn to access your True Essence. You need to realign. You must learn to love and accept yourself. Empathy and forgiveness are essential to this process.

Many therapies embrace this approach. It is important to empathize with yourself, not criticize. I believe that criticism is the most stressful thing you can do or have done to you. It's the epitome of "Don't be yourself." This was a major message in *Doctor's Orders: Go Fishing.*

I learned what most people want is peace of mind. And when I thought about when we have it and how to get it, I realized that it comes largely when we're "going fishing" (doing what we really love). But, remember, people found this too selfish. This was their shadow and inner critic at work. They came to believe that everyone else should come first. You don't get peace of mind running around trying to please everyone. That will get you crazy since everyone has at least a little different idea about most everything. Even religions can't agree on what's right!

So, whenever you find yourself becoming stressed, or your buttons are being pushed, take time as soon as possible to sit down and get in touch with that part of yourself that's feeling out of sorts. Be in touch with your feelings. Don't judge them or try to change them. Treat yourself like you would a best friend. If a best friend were struggling and asked for your help, ideally you wouldn't judge or try to change this person. You would be there for your friend. And whatever it took, you would stay by your friend. That's what you need to do for yourself. I call it loving yourself. You need to learn to accept and love yourself just like you accept and love best friends. You can see their warts and foibles, and you love them just the same. Similarly, be there for yourself. Do this for yourself. Love yourself.

I believe that self-love or loving yourself is the core issue that underlies all of our concerns. This is the same as knowing who you truly are: one with God or Divine Source. For if you really understand that you are one with God, and if you love God, then you must also love yourself. I used to joke that if I could create a new diagnostic code for physical or mental disorders, it would be called "Forgotten Identity." We have forgotten the truth of who we are, and this loss of connection to our Essential Nature causes or contributes to a breakdown in our health. We must stop the self-criticism, and learn to forgive ourselves for not living up to some learned, arbitrary ideal that came from our parents, community, or culture.

Anthropology is the scientific study of human nature and behavior. And what it tells us is that all of our most closely cherished beliefs about ourselves are learned. Whatever you believe to be right or wrong, there was a time somewhere in history that someone else believed exactly the opposite. For example, every role and trait that you may ascribe to males, at one time in history has been the moral and socially approved role for females.

When I was a university graduate student I wrote and published an article in the journal, *Counseling and Values* titled, "The Suppression of Women by Religion: Implications for Counseling." I was surprised to find how much evidence exists documenting that many religions and societies historically revered women as deities. For thousands of years in recorded history, societies were commonly matriarchal, where women were considered equal to or superior to men. As far back as 7,000 B.C. to 25,000 B.C. many people worshipped a supreme *female* creator! Obviously, this belief changed with the advent of "civilization" and more patriarchal and male-superior reform religions.

Pre-birth Planning

It is very important and very helpful to examine closely and honestly what we believe and why. A unique perspective regarding learning to love ourselves comes from Robert Schwartz and his book, *Your Soul's Plan*. He contends that we plan the vast majority of our life challenges before birth for the purpose of personal growth. Based on his very personal transcendent experience (which I discuss at length in the next chapter), he suddenly knew that life was rich with purpose. Love is who we are. Our soul chose to leave the nonphysical or spiritual realm in order to experience the feelings and emotions that are generated by life in a physical dimension.

Sorrow, pain, and fear do not exist in the spiritual, higher vibrational planes. There we only know ourselves as being joy, peace, and love. "Unqualified compassion and empathy are our very nature." The experience of contrasting emotions on the physical plane allows us and teaches us to learn and experience more fully who we are (love), by experiencing who we are not (fear). If you were treated with a lack of compassion, you would come to appreciate compassion more deeply. A prisoner of war is going to appreciate freedom more fully. "It is the absence of something that best teaches its value and meaning." He says:

> Picture, if you will, a world in which there is only light. If you never experienced darkness, how well would you comprehend and appreciate light? It is the contrast between light and dark that leads to a richer

understanding and, ultimately, a remembering. The physical plane provides us with this contrast because it is one of duality: up and down, hot and cold, good and bad. The sorrow in duality allows us to better know joy. The chaos of Earth enhances our appreciation of peace. The hatred we may encounter deepens our understanding of love. If we never experienced these aspects of humanity, how would we know our divinity?

Pre-birth, pre-scripted life challenges provide us "with a deepened understanding of the compassion, empathy, and oneness that we temporarily screened from our own awareness." Our physical life is the opportunity to "apply, test, and enhance" this understanding. Schwartz states:

Life challenges give us the opportunity to express and thus know ourselves more deeply as love in all its many facets: empathy, forgiveness, patience, nonjudgement, courage, balance, acceptance, and trust. Our earthly experience of ourselves as love may also take the form of understanding, serenity, faith, willingness, gratitude, and humility, among other virtues.

This is why we are here. This is why empathy and forgiveness are essential. We have forgotten who we are. We need to empathize with ourself and each other as we experience "contrast" and negative emotions. Even though we chose to do this pre-birth, we have had this knowledge screened from our awareness. We can become very immersed in the physical. You will remember when I used to tell myself and my patients that life stinks, as part of trying to make sense of suffering.

We've chosen to experience fear-based emotions, ones that contrast with love on purpose in order to grow in our understanding of love. Where we might be prone to say that we need to forgive ourselves for not being perfect, we need to forgive ourselves for forgetting that we already are perfect. We need to tell ourselves that we're doing the best we can given the circumstances.

You Did The Best You Could

I'd like to introduce a little logic and a practical reason for forgiveness, for yourself and others. I'm going to make up a story to help make my point.

There was a boy who was a really good basketball player. He loved to play the game. One day, at the very end of a game, the score was tied. And this boy attempted a last-second shot that would have won the game. But he missed. He felt really bad. But because he was fouled in the act of shooting, he would get two foul shots. If he makes one, the game's over, and his team wins. He stepped to the line, and shot the first foul shot, and missed. Again, he felt terrible – for himself, and that he was letting down his team and a gym full of fans. Then the other team called a time-out to "ice the shooter." They hoped that he would become more tense about the pressure of having to make this next foul shot by taking the time-out. Hopefully, he would miss again. So, the teams went to their benches. Image how this boy felt.

Now I'd like you to imagine you're the coach of this boy who just missed the last two shots, and has one more that can win the game. When he comes to the bench, what are you going to do or say to this boy? Would you berate the boy for having missed the two shots? Would you remind the team about any earlier times in the game where they might have played better so that they wouldn't have found themselves in this position? Probably you would want to focus strictly on the present moment. The only thing that matters is the next shot. Would you want to give energy to anything other than on making the next shot? It would make no sense to focus on past shortcomings. As the coach, you would likely say something like, "OK, we gotta' regroup. Here's what we gotta' do." And you would have the team totally focused on what it will take to move forward and win the game.

And, so, now as you appreciate this story, and the need to focus on what you want, not what you don't want in your life, you may remember a time when you felt you let someone down, or didn't measure up to someone's expectations. Or you did it to someone else. And as you remember a time in your life, hopefully you can find yourself fully empathetic with yourself or them for feeling the discomfort, anxiety, pain or shame of someone's disapproval. You realize that it wasn't anyone's fault. *You did the best you could at the time*. Here's the new game plan: 1) Own your feelings. Take responsibility for, and love and accept your feelings. 2) Empathize with yourself (or others), 3) Forgive yourself (or others), 4) Go for it! (Focus only on what you want). Go fishing.

Remember "the power of now." The only thing that matters is this moment. It does no good whatsoever to drag up the past. Is that going to help you get what you want?

Besides the point of focusing on what you want, and not wasting time or energy or doing anything other than what's going to help you get what you want (make the next shot), consider this. Remember that thoughts and feelings are energy and have real consequences. If you are harboring any negative thoughts toward others, you in fact will hurt yourself more than them. The original blueprint of your negativity is in your mind, and affects you more than it could possibly hurt another. Do not give others that power over you. The fact is that the people who seem to hurt you the most can only hurt you if you let them. Obviously, this will take awareness and discipline.

This reminds me of one of my favorite stories. A man would buy a newspaper each day from a newspaper stand. The man who sold the paper was always gruff, but the man purchasing the paper was always pleasant. One day a friend was with the man while he was getting his paper, and he observed how kind his friend was, while the vendor was anything but pleasant. As they walked away, the friend asked, "Why were you so nice when that guy was such a creep?" The friend responded, "I guess I never want anyone else to decide how I should act." Who do you want to determine how you should act? Who do you want to control you and how you want to be? Or feel?

Another suggestion is that you could use your emotions at this time to "charge" your new thought pattern of what you do want. Use your disappointment, anger, shame or pain to strengthen the outcome you want. When you find yourself upset about something, as soon as possible, with all of your emotion, scream to yourself, "The next shot absolutely goes in."

You could also use your emotions as yet another way to remind yourself to refocus on what you want. The next time you're feeling out of sorts, tell your feelings, "Thank you for reminding me that we're not doing this anymore."

Of course, reflecting back on the last chapter and oneness: Whatever you do affects everything and everyone. Sometimes a great motivator for people to not get stuck in negative thoughts and feelings is to remember that their emotional state is not only being broadcast through their own body, but out into the universe. Remember how this affects the weather? It can contribute to prosperity or famine, harmony or discord, war or peace. Here's my mantra: I signed up. I show up. I shine my light.

There is a very practical reason to love your enemies. Loving thoughts and behavior beget more love. Hateful, depressive, and angry thoughts beget more of that. Revenge is your worst enemy. Unless your idea of revenge is to tell the people who bug you the most that you love them. It's a great way to refocus from negative thinking. And a warped humorous upside to this is that it will drive them crazy. Think about it.

Whenever you're feeling fearful in any way, subconsciously a part of you is feeling vulnerable, and wants to feel safe and loved. As you learned as children to feel ashamed for not being good or doing what's right, or letting your parents down, you learned to think less of yourself and that maybe you're not worth loving. You then looked for someone or something to make you feel good about yourself. And this is the root of addictive behaviors: You're going to do whatever you need to do to find self-respect and a feeling of connectedness or belonging. Or you'll do whatever necessary to numb or repress these feelings of low self-worth and the shame and pain of feeling unloved.

My addictions were, and to some extent still are, food, sports, women, and sex. Until somewhat recently, as I became more aware of what I'm trying to pass along to you, I looked to these to feel good about myself. It's like the idea of looking for love in all the wrong places. I needed to realize that these addictions were temporary fixes, but weren't going to be deeply soul satisfying or healthy. My wife is my greatest teacher.

There's a definite part of me that doesn't want to be married. It's really about fear of intimacy, and my own issues of trust and self-worth. But it took me a while to figure that out. Excuse a bit of a digression, but I want to give you a clearer idea of my aversion to marriage. Approximately 30 years ago, I was lecturing about relationships and marriage. Only instead of saying the word "marriage", I said "funeral". Talk about a Freudian slip! I didn't get married until I was 51 years old. I always thought that I was protecting my independence. Of the many relationships I've had, I never really saw that maybe I had something to do with my relationships not lasting more than about two years.

I actually was engaged to be married when I was 45 to an oncology nurse specialist. She was terrific and a lot of things I'm not in some ways, which I found very attractive. She was spontaneous, creative, intelligent, in touch with her feelings, communicative, flexible, fun, genuine, and spiritual. She even had a doctorate in nursing and a Masters Degree of Divinity. It seemed like a great fit. At first. But, of course, I found ways (subconsciously) to sabotage this relationship like every other one I'd been in. My fear of intimacy, and not loving myself, would rear their ugly heads and be expressed as self-centeredness and any number of insecurities. Even though I was a psychologist, and should have known better, she helped me see that I was a terrible listener and partner. And I didn't have a clue.

When she broke off the engagement, I finally decided that maybe I had something to do with it, and that I needed to seriously reassess myself. I came to realize that my learned sense of maleness and being the king of the beasts wasn't going to cut it. I then practiced guided imagery daily to prepare myself for a loving, lasting relationship.

The next year I met Shelly, who became my best friend for years before we married. In fact, we never dated. We were together most of the time, but not romantically. The thing I liked most about her was how non-threatening she was. She really liked and respected me, and was fun to be with. And she had this pure heart.

At some point she revealed her interest in having a relationship with me beyond our friendship. I was not ready for this. Fortunately she was *very* patient with me, and I grew into realizing that she would be an ideal partner. However, this does not mean this went smoothly. The good news was that I was truly committed to making this relationship and marriage work. But without her unbelievable love and patience, I would have sabotaged this one, too.

She has helped me look at and resolve the anger I've held related to my father's strict discipline and my prime-time self-centeredness. I honestly usually think of

myself first. Maybe this is why I'm so motivated to teach
others to identify and meet their needs. But in learning to
love my wife, and our commitment to our marriage, I am
finally learning to accept and love myself. I still love
food, Penn State wrestling and football, and sex, but I
have a very different understanding and perspective.

Earlier in 2008 I read the book *Radical Forgiveness*
by Colin Tipping, and attended his Radical Forgiveness
workshop with my wife. He stressed that our life is
always reflected in our beliefs. If you were to make a list
of the things you really dislike in another, these are in fact
what you have not been able to accept about yourself.
You attract people so you can project onto them. Shelly
really liked Colin's statement, "You spot it: You got it!"
What you see in others is being mirrored back to you.
These are the very things you need to heal and love about
yourself. As Robert Schwartz says in *Your Soul's Plan*:

> ...There is a part of ourselves we
> judge as weak. If we did not see ourselves
> as weak at certain times or under certain
> circumstances, then it would be impossible
> to hold that judgment of someone else.
> Instead, either we would not notice the
> behavior or traits that we view as weakness,
> or we would not see those behaviors and
> traits as weakness. All judgment of others is
> cloaked self-judgment.

People who push our buttons are blessings in
disguise. They give us opportunities to get in touch with
our original pain, and to see beliefs about ourselves so
that we can heal and grow. Subconsciously and

energetically we attract what we need to balance in our lives. It is not about trying to change ourselves, but learning to accept and love ourselves just the way we are.

Rather than blame or judge others, we need to forgive them and be grateful for them. These are opportunities to discover the truth of who we really are. Actually, we need to forgive ourselves for creating the situation in the first place. Remember the law of attraction. We drew them to us. And, although this might sound a bit philosophical or theoretical, there's really no one to forgive. There's only one of us: God appearing in different forms. In the end it's about your soul's journey and deepest desire to reconnect with its Source. It's about realizing your full potential, understanding love more fully, and finding your way back home, where only love abides.

As Colin says, the reason we get upset is because someone resonates within ourselves the things that we've disowned, denied, repressed, and projected onto them. They're simply reflecting what we need to love and accept within ourselves. "This concept – *what we attract and judge in others is really what we condemn in ourselves* – is … the key to our own soul-level healing." The part of ourselves that we have rejected is crying out to be accepted. "It acknowledges that the Divine essence within, the knowing part of yourself, your soul – whatever you want to call it, has set the situation up for you, so you can learn, grow and heal a misperception or a false belief." We're all "doing a healing dance" with each other.

I also like the way Gregg Braden explains mirroring in his book, *The Divine Matrix*:

> ... The Divine Matrix works like a great cosmic screen that allows us to see the nonphysical energy of our emotions and beliefs (our anger, hate, and rage; as well as our love, compassion, and understanding) projected in the physical medium of life.
>
> Just as a movie screen reflects without judgment the image of whatever or whoever has been filmed, the Matrix appears to provide an unbiased surface for our inner experiences and beliefs to be seen in the world.

Quantum physics research and many spiritual disciplines describe a unified field of consciousness or what's also called, the zero point field. Our thoughts and feelings act as disturbances or interruptions in this field. When we disturb the tranquility of this field through any thoughts and feelings that suggest separation vs. oneness with this Divine Matrix, it interrupts the natural flow or beingness of this perfect harmonious state. This leads to a breakdown in the physical. So, whether or not you're consciously aware of your thoughts and feelings, they are constantly affecting your life circumstances and health. Knowing this, we can use this knowledge purposefully to create what we want in our lives.

A major message in Gregg Braden's books, *The Isaiah Effect, Secrets of the Lost Mode of Prayer, The Divine Matrix*, and *The Spontaneous Healing of Beliefs* is that, "Feeling is the language that speaks to the Divine Matrix". He beckons us to "Feel as though our goal is accomplished and our prayer is already answered." Gregg discovered this while on a pilgrimage into Tibet. An abbot of one of the monasteries said to him very simply that whatever rituals they may perform as part of their extensive daily prayerful activities, that "Feeling is the prayer!"

This supports well my study of guided imagery. It is important to imagine and immerse yourself in the "end result." As Jesus states in Mark 11:24, "Therefore I tell you, whatever you ask for in prayer, believe that you have received it, and it will be yours." Whatever you're wanting or praying for, it is important to act as if you've already received it. It becomes a prayer of gratitude, knowing that God or the zero point field instantaneously responds to your every request, thought, and feeling.

Four books that I'd like to recommend that I found very inspirational in my search to understand guided imagery and the power of the mind are, *The Neville Reader: A Collection of Spiritual Writings and Thoughts on Your Inner Power to Create an Abundant Life* by Neville Goddard, *The Man Who Tapped the Secrets of the Universe* by Glenn Clark, *Life and Teaching of the Masters of the Far East* by Baird Spalding, and *Ask and It Is Given* by Esther and Jerry Hicks. As much as anyone I've known or read about, Neville understood and lived his beliefs in prayer as "the art of *believing*". Glenn Clark tells the story about Dr. Walter Russell, who truly lived and inspired the inherent genius that lies within us all. Baird Spalding was part of a research party that visited the Far East in 1894. His books detail his experiences while living among the Great Masters of the Himalayas. He came away convinced that these adepts knew a truer, deeper self, that which we call God, and that this God within was literally omnipotent. He learned that we all have unlimited power to perform what we might normally call miracles. And *Ask and It Is Given* is simply the Bible of how to use your thoughts and feelings to make all of your dreams come true. Esther and Jerry Hicks (and Abraham) speak eloquently, clearly, and forcefully about the law of attraction, and that there is nothing you cannot have or do.

Loving Yourself

Earlier I noted that the disorder of "Forgotten Identity" is the core issue that underlies all of our concerns. We have forgotten who we truly are and our Divine connection. If we knew and lived this fundamental truth, surely we would love ourselves enough that we would take care of ourselves better. We would understand our true self-worth and live accordingly. This is where I want to reemphasize the three pillars of wellness: nutrition, exercise, and stress management. Love yourself enough to address these areas of your life. The 2008 book, *Blue Zones*, by Dan Buettner is an excellent reminder how important this is – if you want to live longer.

Dan Buettner was asked to write a cover story for *National Geographic* magazine about the "Secrets of Long Life." This took him to places all over the world, which came to be called "Blue Zones", where people lived the longest, healthiest lives. The premise of these population studies is that if you want to add at least ten good years to your life, optimize your lifestyle. It's about environment, outlook, lifestyle, and food, - not your genes. In conjunction with the National Institute on Aging, this is what they concluded were the lessons for living longer:

1. Move naturally. Engage in fun activities. Be active without having to think about it. An ideal routine would include a combination of aerobic, balancing, and muscle-strengthening activities 30-60 minutes daily.
2. Cut calories by 20%. Stop eating when your stomach is 80% full.
3. Avoid meat and processed foods. Eat more fruits, vegetables, and nuts.
4. Drink red wine in moderation.
5. Have a strong sense of purpose, a goal in life – why you want to wake up in the morning. Be fully immersed in what you're doing.
6. Take time to relieve stress: rest, socialize, and meditate.
7. Participate in a spiritual community.
8. Make family, togetherness, and support a priority.
9. Surround yourself with those who share these Blue Zone values. This reinforces good habits, mutual support, and social connectedness.

Costa Rica, one of these Blue Zones, spends only 15% as much money on healthcare compared to the United States. Yet they are living longer, healthier lives than people anywhere else on earth. Nutrition, exercise, a sense of fulfillment and being valued and cared for – this is their prescription for a good life. "It's about loving and being loved."

I want to add here what may be a bit of a digression, but if you want to get a sense of what it means to be fully alive, read the book, *To Reach The Clouds*, by Philippe Petit. Or view the movie or DVD about him, *Man On Wire*.

Philippe Petit pulled off what may be the "artistic crime of the century". One day he was flipping through a magazine, and saw the plans to construct the Twin Towers in New York City. As crazy as this is about to sound, he drew a line between these two tallest skyscrapers in the world, and "knew" that he had to walk on a tightrope between them. On August 7, 1974, after years of planning, cunning, scheming, you name it, he walked back and forth on a metal cable eight times, nearly 45 minutes, between the towers of the World Trade Center!

While his story is about daring and mastery, it's an inspiration for all who want to achieve their wildest dreams. His life and his story are pure poetry. While you may think him insane or at least crazy, I am certain he was living his connection to Divine Source. If you watch the DVD, be sure to see the "Special Features" and his interview discussing his life and how singly focused he was on living his joy and passion. He is a great example of what it means to "go fishing", and to follow your bliss. Live your truth. Go for it!

Chapter 7 - Love and Healing

When my wife and I moved to southern Oregon in 2006 I first began to work with a progressive nursing and rehabilitation center in Grants Pass. Immediately I called around the area offering to speak about wellness and mind-body medicine. When I phoned Rogue Valley Medical Center, I was referred to Dr. Robin Miller, who was the Medical Director of Triune Integrative Medicine, which was affiliated with the medical center.

Robin was intrigued with my background and training, and we set up an appointment to meet. She said that she was looking for someone to do guided imagery work and maybe also work with her cancer patients at Triune. I had to laugh at the coincidence of Robin's interests and my credentials. Robin had trained with Dr. Andrew Weil at the University of Arizona's integrative medicine program. What synchronicity that at that time I was co-authoring the chapter on mind-body medicine in his new book, *Integrative Oncology*.

Leonard Laskow

Soon after I began working at Triune, Robin told me about Dr. Leonard Laskow, who had a special interest in love and healing. Len had been speaking to Robin's husband, who also is a physician, and when he mentioned this to Robin, she was sure that I would like to meet him. She was so right.

It just so happened that Len was soon to be speaking in the area, and I arranged to attend his lecture on "Healing with Love," which was the title of his book. After I heard him speak, and when I reviewed the material that he handed out to the audience, I couldn't have been more interested in him and his work. I was compelled to meet and talk with him further, and, fortunately, he agreed to meet me for lunch. When he heard about my work and current book, *Why Love Heals*, he offered to support me. I've since attended a number of his seminars. After he heard me speak at Triune about the Law of Attraction, he asked if we could set up a full-day workshop, which we then co-presented in the spring of 2008 in Ashland, Oregon. I'm pleased to say that we have become good friends, and he remains a great inspiration for me.

In his book, *Healing With Love*, Len states:

> Every structure, animate or inanimate, has a set of energetic vibrations or frequencies that are unique and natural to it. When a structure is vibrating in a way that is characteristic for it, it is said to be in resonance. That resonant frequency, or set of frequencies, is the tune to which it dances best. ...
>
> In the presence of a coherent magnetic field, such as that produced by MRI, the hydrogen protons spin in concert as they align themselves with the field. In effect, they all dance the same dance; they become one. Similarly, when you create a coherent loving field, everything within that field begins to vibrate as one, to dance to the same rhythm.

When all begins to vibrate as one, separation disappears and there is only oneness... In this state of oneness, the natural order and harmony inherent in the tissues, cells, molecules, atoms, and subatomic particles reassert themselves. The cells remember the higher order and balance of health and wholeness. Love is their reminder...If we view love as a universal pattern of resonant energy, we begin to recognize it as an energetic pattern that can influence other energies to move toward wholeness and healing. Our universe can be thought of as a matrix of consciousness that emerged out of the void. Love is the connecting glue of unifying consciousness in the universe and is ever-present whether we are aware of it or not.

I want to take time here to say more about Len and his work and research regarding love and healing, specifically with the use of intention and imagery. The opening sentences in his book, *Healing With Love*, state, "Healing occurs naturally, and love heals. We can use our thoughts, our hands, our hearts, and our higher consciousness to facilitate healing." After 25 years of practice as a medical doctor he became convinced "that the physician only treats; it is nature that does the actual healing... the natural impulse of life is to heal itself." The constant in all healing was:

    ...the presence of someone to facilitate the natural healing processes, to

> focus attention on and encourage the patient
> toward recovery. In other words, the active
> ingredient was not surgery, antibiotics, or
> other mechanical methods. Rather, it was
> love: the impulse toward unity,
> nonseparation, and wholeness.

You can see how well Len's work agrees with my premise that health requires that we align all aspects of ourselves with our spiritual essence. And why love heals.

Len had a curiosity for various healing approaches, and a personal interest in meditation. One day while he was on a retreat and in a deep meditation, he had a sense of being filled with light, and an inner voice said, "Your work is to heal with love." This experience led him to investigate further how love literally could affect a healing response. He found that non-ordinary states of consciousness, like meditation, had many benefits, including improved health.

Len had a good friend and colleague at Stanford University, who was a neurobiologist, Dr. Glen Rein. Together they conducted several experiments to test the effectiveness of intention and imagery while in a meditative state that Len called a "loving healing presence."

In one of their studies they tested the impact of thought vs. imagery on the growth rate of cancer cells. In this case Len literally held a Petri dish of cancer cells and projected the thought to the cells, "Return to the natural order and growth rate of your pre-cancerous cell line." This produced an 18% inhibition in their cell growth. Then when he held that thought coupled with the specific image of a reduced number of cancer cells, there was a

39% reduction of cells in the culture. Adding specific imagery to thought, while in a "loving resonance with the cells," doubled the effectiveness of intention.

Glen and Len later tested modulating the molecular confirmation of DNA. They found that Len could wind or unwind human placental DNA by entering into a loving state, and using thought and imagery! The Institute of HeartMath invited Glen and Len to their laboratory to explore this further.

The Institute of HeartMath is a research and educational organization that has explored extensively the physiological and emotional connections between the heart and brain. They have found consistently that negative emotions create disorder in the heart's rhythms and the autonomic nervous system, which leads to increased stress within the body. This chronic fight-or-flight response leads to disease. They were pleased to find that Glen and Len's "loving resonance" approach could affect a more harmonious bodily state.

Using an electrocardiogram, electroencephalogram, and electromyologram to monitor Len's meditative state, they found that he produced a remarkable state of internal coherence. With loving, focused intention he was able to unwind the double helix of DNA. When they looked at the frequency power spectrum of other people who had no special meditative training, but were "trying to love," there was a lack of coherence that Len had been able to achieve.

The importance of coherence, by example, is that coherence is what makes a laser light so powerful. The waves of the laser beam are in-phase or in sync, functioning in harmony and with maximum efficiency. In comparison, the filament in an ordinary light bulb emits light that has no fixed phase relationship, and is therefore distorted and unfocused. Len proposed that when you enter a loving state of consciousness (cardiac coherence as measured by the above technology), whatever you focus your attention on guides and amplifies the thought wave. Your persistent focused attention on a desired outcome while in a coherent state is a very focused energy that has the ability to create or transform. This potentially explains the passages in the Bible (Revised Standard Version): "For truly, I say to you, if you have faith as a grain of mustard seed, you will say to this mountain, 'Move hence to yonder place,' and it will move; and nothing will be impossible to you" (Matthew 17:20). And in Luke 17:6, "And the Lord said, 'If you had faith as a grain of mustard seed, you could say to this sycamore tree, 'Be rooted up, and be planted in the sea, and it would obey you."

The Institute of HeartMath has demonstrated consistently and convincingly that when you become more balanced mentally and emotionally your health improves. This is documented well in the book, *The HeartMath Solution.*

In 1995, Dr. Rollin McCraty and colleagues at the Institute of HeartMath published an article titled, "The effects of emotions on short-term power spectrum analysis of heart rate variability" in the *American Journal of Cardiology.* They demonstrated that negative emotions, such as anger, created "jagged and distorted" heart rhythms. Positive emotions, such as gratitude and appreciation, increased order and balance in the nervous system, producing smooth, harmonious heart rhythms. Additional research led to techniques where research subjects were able to create a state of inner balance and harmony at will. When you focus on feelings such as happiness, compassion, love, appreciation and care, your heart rhythms become more coherent, which "affects virtually every organ in the body".

The Institute of HeartMath has been a leader in this research. In 1995, Glen Rein and colleagues published an article titled, "The physiological and psychological effects of compassion and anger" in the *Journal of Advancement in Medicine*. This groundbreaking study tested the impact of one five-minute segment of time spent recalling something that made the test subjects angry compared to five minutes of focusing on feeling care and compassion. The five-minute memory of anger impaired the effectiveness of their immune system for over six hours. After five minutes of feeling care and compassion, the subjects had an immediate 41% average increase in an antibody called secretory IgA, which is a first line of defense against invading pathogens, and is a measure of immune system health. After one hour their IgA levels returned to normal, but then slowly increased over the next six hours.

This research epitomizes the findings of quantum physics. When you align yourself with the energy matrix of harmony and order that underlies all of physical matter, you become more coherent. Coherence means no energy is wasted. Power is maximized. There is no stress or resistance. And, as a result, the underlying quantum field of energy now flows through your body maximizing its function. Love shifts the body from a fight-or-flight stress response to one of order and calm.

Love has a universal frequency and expresses the innate harmony of the universe. It is the common frequency of everything. It is the Divine Matrix. We, as consciousness, in connection with Divine Source, are the Divine Matrix and the Divine Creator. And our health, our relationships, and the world we live in are all a reflection of our beliefs. One of the clearest indicators of how well you are aligned with this "zero point field," the vast quantum field that connects everything, is indeed, to look at your health.

Spirituality and Health

Dr. Deepak Chopra was one of the first to popularize this understanding in his many books, including *Quantum Healing: Exploring the Frontiers of Mind/Body Medicine*. He presented evidence how "positive visualizations" and the "will to live" could produce spontaneous remissions. His study of the ancient Ayurveda healing tradition revealed what quantum physics and related research was now discovering: "that the human body is controlled by a 'network of intelligence' grounded in quantum reality." When we are in harmony with it, our physiology changes and our health improves. When we are out of tune with our Essential Nature, sickness results. Our thoughts and feelings and the cells of our body are connected "with the fundamental units of matter and energy."

A cardinal belief of Ayurvedic medicine is that the body is created out of consciousness. Healing is primarily a mental process, not a physical one. Chopra states:

> In my own practice, several cancer patients have recovered completely after being pronounced incurable and given only a few months to live. I didn't think they

were miracles; I thought they were proof that the mind can go deep enough to change the very patterns that design the body. It can wipe mistakes off the blueprint, so to speak, and destroy any disease – cancer, diabetes, coronary heart disease – that has disturbed the design.

Sri Swamini Mayatitananda, who is often referred to as Mother or Mother Maya, has authored three books on Ayurveda including, *Ayurveda: A Life of Balance* written in 1994. Using her pen name Maya Tiwari, she has sold more than a million copies. Following a terminal diagnosis of ovarian cancer, and given only a few months to live, she received healing information from her deceased father during periods of meditation. He told her that she needed to reconnect spiritually. She claims that opening her inner awareness to the Divine, and following ancient Ayurvedic traditions, led to her cure. She went on to open the Wise Earth School of Ayurveda to teach what she calls, "inner medicine." Catherine Elliott Escobedo describes this approach in her Winter 2008-2009 article, "The Everyday Miracle of Healing: A Profile of Mother Maya" in the *Shift* quarterly by the Institute of Noetic Sciences. She lists the following principles on which "inner medicine" is based:

- *Wholeness: Realizing the true self to be one with nature*
- *Simplicity: Practicing humility through surrender to nature's intelligence*
- *Harmony: Committing to harmony within and without*

- *Memory: Restoring cosmic, cognitive, and ancestral memories*
- *Rhythm: Honoring   nature's nourishment in food, breath, and sound*
- *Sacred Practice: Aligning every activity in accord with nature's rhythms*
- *Consciousness: Cultivating   inner awareness*

Perhaps the greatest example of the embodiment of the world's great spiritual principles is taught at the Oneness University in India. Founded by Sri Amma and Bhagavan in 2002, it is estimated that they have more than 100 million followers. Their aim is to put all people in touch with the truth of their faith. They believe that the nature of existence is bliss, and that spirituality is about happiness. When you have a direct experience of oneness, not just beliefs or words, no one will need to be taught virtue or love; it will become your natural state. There is an emphasis on self-acceptance and discovering love within yourself. There is only one cause for human problems – the sense of separateness from God, the one life that is expressing itself in all forms. An excellent description of their work is in the book, *Awakening Into Oneness* by Arjuna Ardagh.

These principles are similar to shamanism, which dates back tens of thousands of years. In his book, *The World of Shamanism*, psychiatrist Dr. Roger Walsh concludes that there are seven spiritual practices that are essential for living life to the fullest: 1) Living ethically, 2) Transforming emotions, 3) Redirecting motivation, 4) Training attention, 5) Refining awareness, 6) Cultivating wisdom, and 7) Serving others.

As I noted earlier, shamanism views disease and related symptoms as an indication of something being out of balance with your natural state of harmony and order. Your symptoms are a form of biofeedback letting you know that you are blocking the natural flow of the Divine Source that is the source of all life. From a spiritual or philosophic perspective, this Life Force or vital energy is a universal concept and has been given many names, such as Holy Spirit, Qi, or Chi, and Prana.

In traditional Chinese medicine, especially acupuncture, it is believed that the human body has energy meridians very similar to the circulatory system. This Qi or life force enters the body through specific acupuncture points. Evidence of this is in research demonstrating a dramatically decreased electrical resistance at acupuncture points compared with points on the skin surrounding it. This life-giving energy flows along these meridians just as blood flows through veins and arteries. Imagine what happens to our health if we have impaired blood circulation. Any block of the flow of this all-pervasive life energy has similar consequences to our health.

So, going back to our earlier discussion of character strengths and virtues, and why these are so revered and valued. It's because they resonate energetically with the quantum field and Divine Source. And we experience a life of greater ease as a result when living these virtues.

In electricity, the term "in phase" means that electricity is flowing with the least amount of resistance, which allows for maximal power. An electrician's ohmmeter is actually recording the resistance of a circuit. In your body, stress is equated with resistance. Any thought or feeling you have that suggests "separation" from the field, or dissonance with the core fact of our oneness with God, creates resistance and results in a diminished flow of life force energy in your body. Love maximizes the flow of this energy. This is why love heals.

The Science of Altruistic Love

In 2001 Dr. Stephen Post began The Institute for Research on Unlimited Love (IRUL) at Case Western Medical School in Cleveland, Ohio. He had taught medical ethics there for many years before. (He and IRUL are now at Stony Brook University in New York). His 2007 book, *Why Good Things Happen to Good People* documents his 25 years of studying generous behavior. Its simple message is, "Give and be happier. Give and be healthier. Give and live longer." The research reviewed in this book is extensive, and clearly demonstrates that gratitude (an aspect of love) has many health benefits. The simple fact is that helping others makes us feel good, and one interesting finding in these studies is that giving support improved health more than receiving it.

Over the past 100 years, about 500 scientific studies demonstrate the power of unselfish love to enhance health. Why is giving good medicine? Post believes it is most likely related to decreasing a stress (fight or flight) response in the body. He states:

> Generous behavior is closely associated with reduced risk of illness and mortality and lower rates of depression. Even more remarkable, giving is linked to traits that undergird a successful life, such as social competence, empathy, and positive

emotion. By learning to give, you become more effective at living itself.

One of the researchers who Post mentions in his book is Dr. Pitirim Sorokin, who established the Harvard Research Center in Creative Altruism after founding the Department of Sociology at Harvard University in 1931. Post wrote the introduction to Sorokin's newly released classic text, *The Ways and Power of Love*, in 2002. He notes that Sorokin's scope and depth of his analysis of love is "uniquely insightful." It's certainly all of that. It is a tome of research and his beliefs about altruistic love, and why the study of love must be included in the empirical sciences. He particularly chides psychology and sociology for their failure to research the nature of love and its practical uses.

What I found especially interesting is how much attention he gives to mystical, religious, and spiritual considerations of love. Sorokin begins his first chapter on "The Religious Aspects of Love" stating that "love is identified with God, the highest value" in all of the great religions. He cites large numbers of "eminent ethical teachers", from Buddha to Jesus to Gandhi and Albert Schweitzer, as factual evidence for the importance of incorporating an understanding of love into science. He similarly cites seemingly every leading thinker in history, from Pythagoras, Socrates, Plato, and Aristotle to Meister Eckhart, Emerson, Tolstoi, Dostoievsky, and many other philosophers, about the role of love, ethics, and God in our lives. In summation, he says that there is remarkable "similarity, even unanimity of the precepts of all ethical systems of love... It cannot be explained away as a mere chance concordance of a number of chance opinions of a number of chance ideologists… For this reason it is an important factual evidence."

Sorokin also discusses one point where he claims all psychiatrists and psychotherapists agree:

> …*that the main curative agent in all the diverse psychiatric techniques is the 'acceptance' of the patient by the therapist, the rapport of empathy, sympathy, kindness, and love established between the therapist and the patient. In other words, the essence of curative therapy consists in the patient's exposure to the "radiation" of understanding, kindness, and love of the therapist…*

Rapport between the therapist and patient is more fundamental than the type of therapy employed. By contrast, any communication that patients perceive to be disrespectful, impersonal, cold, and unsupportive is the "worst and least effective therapy." Sorokin is adamant about "love in all its various forms" being "the real curative agent in mental disease." However, he acknowledges that it is advisable that love be guided by adequate scientific training. He then cites psychologist, Dr. Carl Rogers, as an exemplary example of the necessary components of therapy (support, security, understanding, acceptance, and warmth).

Roger's therapy is often referred to as "client-centered" therapy, and is credited for having profound influences on both individual and group counseling. His theory of personality is significant in his emphasis on the basic qualities of the individual. All theories of personality postulate about the nature of human beings to some extent. However, Rogers consistently emphasized the dignity and worth of each person. What I found especially noteworthy in my university studies was his belief that people have a natural capacity for growth and development beyond their intellect or socialization. The individual is basically good, and will develop satisfactorily if given the opportunity and support in dealing with the stresses of life. The person has an innate self-actualizing tendency.

At the end of my doctoral program in psychology, I was required to write my own theory of personality. I remember discussing this with the dean of the graduate school, and how neither of us was very comfortable with this belief in an innate (which means unlearned) tendency of the individual. Didn't this have to be learned or acquired somewhere at sometime? Aren't people born with a blank slate, and doesn't their socialization and learned beliefs form their person? Rogers and his inborn self-actualizing qualities were revolutionary to psychology when introduced, and I have to admit that decades later science continues to struggle with this.

I propose that this is another example of "forgotten identity." Rogers may not have expressed his spiritual beliefs in his academic and clinical approach to psychology, but he demonstrated a clear understanding of the goodness and God-ness of the individual in his own right. Science has largely resisted any links to spirituality. It has been slow to accept a mind-body relationship, let alone a mind-body-spirit approach to well-being. This has been my own journey in learning why love heals.

Of course it wasn't acceptable in my scientific training and studies to allow for a spiritual perspective.

And I didn't know much at all about quantum physics then either. But I hope that it is becoming clear that metaphysics and quantum physics have been, and are in, strong agreement: The core of who we are is love, harmony, and order. And, indeed, it is our learned beliefs upon birth that allow or thwart this natural state to emerge and prosper. Just as Rogers said that we have this natural tendency to grow and develop, quantum physics claims that the quantum field, which encompasses and connects everything, has a natural drive toward coherence. Metaphysical systems profess that Truth naturally seeks and finds its way through all creation: We are innate perfection, one with God, and have infinite power that invariably prevails.

Bedside Manner

Larry Dossey embodies for me the qualities of "eminent ethical teachers" as described by Professor Sorokin. He has been a guiding light and more than a pioneer in mind-body-spirit medicine. As a physician he has been an extremely valuable voice in asking science and medical practice to look at the scientific and ethical reasons to adopt what he calls "Era III" medicine. He says this needs to encompass the use of "physicalistic" medicine, including drugs, surgery, and radiation (what he calls Era I). It also needs to incorporate emotions, the placebo effect, stress management, psychosomatic disease, complementary or alternative medicine, and what in general has come to be called mind-body medicine approaches (Era II). Era III medicine additionally includes spirituality or consideration of nonlocality, and addresses more directly the doctor-patient relationship. It is this relationship that Sorokin claimed was the essence of any curative therapy. It requires empathy or what is called the doctor's "bedside manner."

There is a classic and often cited article titled, "The Care of the Patient" by Dr. Francis W. Peabody in the *Journal of the American Medical Association* (1927). He states that physicians "have been taught a great deal about the mechanism of disease, but very little about the practice of medicine – or, to put it more bluntly, they are too 'scientific' and do not know how to take care of patients." He claims, "the diagnosis and treatment of disease is only one limited aspect of medical practice." Caring for the "emotional life" of the patient can do more "than a book full of drugs." "One of the essential qualities of the clinician is interest in humanity, for the secret of the care of the patient is caring for the patient".

Several studies now show that a strong doctor-patient relationship literally contributes to improved health outcomes. Journalist Maggie Mahar, who specializes in health care, reports on this in an article, "Whatever Happened to Bedside Manner?" on her website (www.healthbeatblog.org):

> A 2005 *Wall Street Journal*/Harris Interactive poll reported that patients' first priority is to have a doctor with strong interpersonal skills: eighty-five percent of Americans said that it was "extremely important" for their doctor to act respectfully toward them, and 84 percent said the same for listening carefully and being "easy to talk to." A 2004 Harris poll of 2,267 U.S. adults found that respondents

cared more that doctors listened to their concerns and questions than they did about doctors being up-to-date on the latest medical research and treatment. And a review of 25 surveys on doctor-patient relationships in a 2001 edition of *The Lancet* said doctors with good bedside manners had a better impact on patients than physicians who were less personal.

The Lancet is one of the world's most highly regarded medical journals. This *Lancet* article by Dr. Zelda Di Blasi and colleagues that was just cited begins by saying, "Throughout history, doctor-patient relationships have been acknowledged as having an important therapeutic effect, irrespective of any prescribed drug or treatment." This review of 25 randomized control trials concludes, "One relatively consistent finding is that physicians who adopt a warm, friendly, and reassuring manner are more effective than those who keep consultations formal and do not offer reassurance." The authors reference other research where "patient and provider expectations may be more important than specific treatment." They note that these "healthcare interactions include factors common to all medical, alternative, and psychological therapies – e.g., attention, bedside manner, empathy, positive regard, compassion, hope, and enthusiasm."

Of course, this isn't just about doctor-patient relationships; it's about all relationships. What relationship wouldn't be improved if we showed attention, empathy, positive regard, hope, and enthusiasm?

I would explain to cancer patients and their families when I taught my classes at the cancer centers that no professional healthcare provider can recommend any treatment approach that isn't researched. (I joked, "Can you spell malpractice?") Ethically and legally, we must base treatment on science. This is all well and good and appropriate. The problem is that we're not doing, or not paying attention to, psycho-social-spiritual research, which common sense says would almost certainly demonstrate the health benefits of loving behavior – for the giver and the receiver. When you resonate with the Truth of who you truly are, harmony and order and good health are the *only* outcome possibilities.

Transcendent Experiences

The fact is that we cannot deny our personal experience just because it isn't supported with research. Dr. David Hufford is Professor Emeritus in the Department of Humanities of Penn State University. His research interests include spirituality, religion, and health. He has authored many papers discussing personal mystical experiences, and how very commonplace they are.

In the book, *The World Was Flooded With Light*, by Genevieve Foster, Hufford writes that these very personal, spiritual experiences are "full of meaning" to the individual who has had such an experience, and that human reason cannot fully comprehend their transcendent nature. As Abraham Maslow states in his book, *Religions, Values, and Peak Experiences,* these experiences are essentially ineffable. Hufford references William James and his classic book, *Varieties of Religious Experience*, which discusses the "noetic" quality of mystical experience. There is a personal "knowing" that is a distinct quality of these "peak experiences." It often involves a sense of oneness, profound love, or loss of the fear of death. James claims that they are "persistent, universal, human experiences."

Hufford notes that there has been a "long-standing academic tendency to explain mystical experience in psychopathological terms," but that "our academic, medical, and religious institutions all have a responsibility to approach this subject more carefully and respectfully than they have in recent years". The academic and medical world "must recognize the existence of spiritual questions as real, complex, and important".

When I worked in State College with the cancer centers, I knew David Hufford because of his affiliation with Penn State and our mutual interest in alternative medicine. I distinctly remember David telling me that mystical experiences were far more common than people realized, had very similar characteristics, and were identified across all cultures worldwide. He said the primary reason he found that people were reluctant to discuss these very personal events was not because they didn't want to appear kooky or mentally unstable. It was because they didn't want their story diminished. They knew their experience was real, and far more meaningful than words could express. My wife has had such an experience.

My wife, Shelly, had been married before for 18 years, when quite unexpectedly her husband died from esophageal cancer. The day he was diagnosed was very troubling and sad. Shelly remembers crying most of the day. That afternoon she walked to the corner grocery store, and on her way home, sobbing continuously, she said that she was stopped in her tracks by an overwhelming feeling of unconditional love. She immediately stopped crying, and was told, "There is something for you to do and your husband's time has come." She told me that she had been very secretive about this experience for the very reason I just mentioned, not wanting her story to be disrespected or misunderstood.

People who have had a near death experience (NDE) are usually similarly concerned about the lessening or dishonoring of their story. I mentioned near death experiences in Chapter 3 regarding the purpose of life. Dr. Moody's research found these experiences to be remarkably similar, consistent, and related to a message of love. The qualities and characteristics of a NDE are so similar to mystical experiences that they tend to be included within the same category of transcendent experiences.

Cardiologist Dr. Pirn van Lommel and his colleagues published research in *The Lancet* in 2001 titled, "Near-death experience in survivors of cardiac arrest: A prospective study in the Netherlands." They reported that between 43% of adults and up to 85% of children who had a life-threatening illness have had a NDE. They concluded that purely physiological, neurophysiological, or psychological factors couldn't explain a NDE. They raised the question, "How could a clear consciousness outside one's body be experienced at that moment that the brain no longer functions during a period of clinical death with flat EEG?" They noted that "NDE pushes at the limits of medical ideas about the range of human consciousness and the mind-brain relation," and that the NDE might be related to a transcendent state of consciousness.

Raymond Moody's first book documenting the NDE, *Life After Life*, has sold more than 15 million copies worldwide. One of the cases that he investigated was Dannion Brinkley, a man who was first struck by lightening in 1975 and apparently died. Dannion tells his story in his best-selling book, *Saved By The Light*. The introduction to this book is written by Moody, who states that Dannion's NDE was one of the most remarkable he has ever heard, including his experience in the "spiritual realm" and the insights and revelations he was given by "Beings of Light".

My wife and I met Dannion when we attended an intuition conference in 1998. Dannion discussed his second NDE that he had in 1989, although interestingly, he was recovering from his third NDE when we met him! What I remember most about first hearing him speak was the story he told about a conversation he had with the surgeon in the hospital who told him that he must have surgery immediately or he would die. Dannion was genuinely thrilled to receive this information. He wanted to die. He knew that you don't die; in fact, his experience was one of a "deep sense of love." Of course, the surgeon thought Dannion was clearly brain-damaged and off his rocker. I laughed hysterically as Dannion described what I could only imagine was an extremely serious moment, and yet ironically of the highest comedy. Please excuse my warped sense of humor, but I don't think I've ever laughed harder.

For those of you who are interested in investigating near death experiences further, I strongly recommend *The Big Book of Near-Death Experiences* written by PMH

Atwater in 2007. She has experienced three NDEs herself, and this is her tenth book on the subject. Her extensive research documents approximately 15 million people have had NDEs, and that consciousness clearly resides beyond the brain and death. I also recommend Mellon-Thomas Benedict and his website (www.mellon-thomas.com). In 1982, Mellon died, succumbing to a terminal cancer diagnosis. Approximately ninety minutes after being pronounced dead, however, he returned to life with a complete remission of the cancer. This is a truly fascinating NDE account where he describes his discovery of "Absolute Pure Consciousness."

How do we resolve our scientific understanding of physical reality with these mystical or transcendent experiences, especially when they're so common and personally meaningful? The January/February (2009) issue of *AARP The Magazine* has an interesting article, "The Mystery of Miracles" by Bill Newcott. Here miracles were defined as an incredible event that cannot be scientifically explained. He reports an AARP survey of 1,300 people aged 45 and over who were asked what they thought about miracles. The results surprised even me. The survey showed that 80% believe in them, 41% believe they happen daily, and 37% claimed to have actually witnessed one. Those who believed, credited the miracles to God, Jesus or the Holy Spirit, angels, saints, relatives or others who are deceased, or other spirits. Only 18% rejected any belief in miracles.

A number of surveys report that at least 90% of Americans believe in God or some Higher Power. This extremely large percentage is not easy to dismiss, nor should it be. Considerable research now exists demonstrating a positive link between spirituality and health. However, I do not believe that physicians or other healthcare professionals should be expected to be expert in spiritual matters. That's what I find so appealing about integrative medicine programs and clinics. Here, specialists from many fields work together offering their expertise. Just as there are many specialists within medicine, and it is common for physicians to refer patients to other medical doctors for specialized treatment, there need to be those on staff who have appropriate training to address these very human, emotional and spiritual issues ethically and legally.

In the 2009 textbook, *Integrative Oncology*, Mary Jo Kreitzer and Ann Marie Dose discuss the relationship between spirituality and health. Their chapter titled, "The Role of Spirituality", reports a number of studies by health professionals regarding the importance of spiritual and religious beliefs and practices:

> A survey of family physicians revealed that 99% believe in the ability of religious beliefs to contribute positively to medical treatment... eighty-seven percent of nurses reported the high importance of paying attention to patients' spiritual needs... [and] 94% of HMO executives indicated that they believe that personal prayer, meditation, or other spiritual and religious practices can speed or help the medical treatment of people who are ill.

Kreitzer and Dose also note that the Joint Commission on Accreditation of Health Organizations (JCAHO) now requires hospitals to add spiritual care to the criteria for accreditation. They also cite a 2006 National Cancer Institute report titled, "Spirituality in Cancer Care," which listed several interventions to address the spiritual concerns of patients. These included recommendations that healthcare providers need skills in listening, being fully present with patients, and the importance of touch. Touch comprised "informal touch provided in usual care," as well as "Therapeutic Touch" and the ancient tradition of "laying on of hands." This NCI report also stated that healthcare providers need ongoing education on commonly used spiritual practices, including prayer; meditation; music, art, and nature; journaling; walking a labyrinth; and spiritual counseling.

For those health professionals who are concerned that they already don't have enough time to attend to their existing busy schedules, I know that adding time to listen and be fully present with patients may sound quite impractical. I'd like to suggest that it's not so much that you need to spend more time – it's about the quality of the time that we spend with patients (or any relationship). Please remember James Lynch's research and the importance of heartfelt communication, even if we have limited time to interact with others.

It is simply no longer acceptable to deny the spiritual and psychological aspects of humanity, and the impact these have on our health and well-being. I believe that an understanding of energy medicine can give us a greater understanding of these issues, which I discuss in the next chapter.

Chapter 8 - Energy Medicine

Indigenous people and ancient wisdom have seemingly always accepted intuition as a way to sense the energy or power of something, and a way to understand the natural world. This usually was infused with their spiritual beliefs. For example, the Chinese approach to medicine has its roots in the spiritual practices of Buddhism and Taoism. Traditional Chinese treatments such as acupuncture, massage, herbs, meditation, and Qi Gong are used to restore balance, and the flow of one's vital energy of "Qi". Qi is believed to be the life force, which animates the body and flows through energy meridians.

Dr. David Eisenberg is an internist in Boston, Massachusetts, on faculty at Harvard Medical School, and director of their integrative medicine program. In 1979, when he was a fourth-year medical student at Harvard, the National Academy of Sciences selected him to be the first United States medical exchange student to China. There he studied at the Beijing College of Traditional Chinese Medicine. He was both fascinated and astounded at how different and effective these "energy medicine" approaches were. Some of his experiences are included in Bill Moyers' book and video, *Healing and the Mind*, a documentary of healing techniques from around the world.

Bill Moyers states in his documentary that he was surprised to see parks full of people in China each day practicing Tai Chi. Tai Chi appears to be a gentle physical exercise type of movement, but these people say that they are feeling and moving energy through their bodies. The philosophy of Tai Chi is that movement and balance are essential for health. By focusing the vital energy Qi in the body, one creates a greater state of balance, which equates with health.

The strangest thing that Bill Moyers reported seeing in China, however, was when an elderly master of martial arts was able to resist the physical strength of several young men. In one instance, at least eight of these young martial arts students attempted to physically push their master teacher at the same time, and could not make him budge. Moyers reported, "It doesn't look real." Indeed it appears very strange to see this older man throw seemingly much stronger and younger men aside without any real physical exertion. But this is a fundamental belief of the martial arts, that one can project a thought, or use one's will, as a kind of energy to affect another person.

For twenty-four centuries, hundreds of millions of Chinese people have practiced different forms of martial arts like Qi Gong. The most widely known in the West is Tai Chi. Many of you probably saw this demonstrated as part of the 2008 Olympic ceremonies in Beijing.

Many claim they can actually "see" and "feel" this flow of energy and where it's blocked. This blocking of the energy results in physical symptoms and illness. Energy medicine approaches claim to restore this flow of energy and, thereby, one's health.

Limited research exists documenting the existence of this Qi energy, but some evidence does support the ability of Qi masters to emit a measurable electromagnetic energy with an ability to affect biological systems. Dr. Beverly Rubik, while at Temple University, did some of this early research. Her book, *Bioelectromagnetics and Energy Medicine: A New Science of Healing*, discusses some of the theory and evidence for this effect. Beverly listed the therapies (such as acupuncture and Therapeutic Touch) that involve subtle biofield interactions that comprise what is called energy medicine. In her paper, *The Biofield Hypotheses: Its Biophysical Basis and Role in Medicine*, supported in part by the National Institutes of Health, she offered a scientific explanation how these therapies involve the transfer of bioinformation. This transfer is carried by a small energy signal that goes beyond the usual molecular concepts of bioinformation. She noted that it is timely for biology to embrace quantum theory. Biologic field concepts such as Burr's L-fields were part of mainstream science for the first half of the twentieth century. As molecular biology became more dominant and developed into big business, a field perspective of life lost prominence. However, the existence of subtle energies has remained central in virtually every indigenous system of medicine, including Oriental medicine, Ayurvedic medicine, modern chiropractic, classic osteopathy, and homeopathy. Rubik believes that the biofield can explain the effectiveness of these ancient medical systems. She cited numbers of more recent scientific studies that support the existence of such a biofield.

An excellent summary of the theory and research of energy medicine is in the book *Vibrational Medicine*, by Dr. Richard Gerber. In his introduction to this book, Dr. Gabriel Cousins describes the human being "as a series of interacting multidimensional energy fields". He claims that the essence of energy medicine approaches, including light and sound, are to rebalance the subtle energies within the body with the introduction of appropriate frequencies or vibrations. It follows, then, that by experiencing love as energy, this would cause the physical body to resonate with a greater state of health and wholeness.

Since everything is energy, including our bodies, then it makes sense that we could and would be affected by other energies. The use of radiation to treat cancer is such an example. But it seems strange to many that one's thoughts or intentions could affect bodily structure or function. Yet there are *hundreds of thousands* of studies demonstrating the therapeutic benefit of hypnosis, biofeedback, guided imagery, and related "intention" approaches. It is hopeful to know that physicians such as Cousins and Gerber consider a person's own harmony and love as an essential part of health and healing. They are rightly and deeply concerned that we have ignored the life force as a subtle energy that animates all of life, the "ghost in the machine," the spiritual dimension. Gerber states in his preface to *Vibrational Medicine*:

> The brain, albeit a complex biocomputer, still needs a programmer to instruct the nervous system how to perform and what acts to accomplish. That conscious entity which uses this biomechanism of the brain and body is the human spirit or soul.

Gerber points out how the discovery of X-rays has capitalized on and developed our understanding of the body as electromagnetic fields. Diagnostic imaging techniques such as CT and PET scans and MRIs are an indispensable part of current medical care. As I just noted, radiation oncologists use electromagnetic radiation to treat cancer. Electrical stimulation, such as a TNS device, is used to control pain and stimulate nerves. Electrotherapy has even been used for tissue regeneration and the healing of fractured bones. Gerber notes:

> *The key principle behind magnetic resonance imaging is the fact that the atoms under study (hydrogen) are being stimulated by the transfer of energy of a specific frequency.* In this case, the energy lies in the realm of radio waves. *The energy is only absorbed by the atom if it is of a particular resonant frequency.*

This is exactly what Len Laskow wrote in his book, Healing With Love, which I mentioned earlier. I want to repeat it here because it is so very relevant to why love heals. Everything and everyone has its own unique vibratory pattern. When that thing or person is vibrating in its natural characteristic way, it functions optimally.

Note that the MRI only absorbs atoms that are of the same frequency or vibratory pattern – when they are in resonance. Our core essence or energy pattern is love. When we experience love, our bodies and being naturally absorb and align with this resonant energy. Health and well-being are the natural consequence of this experience. This is why love heals.

David Eisenberg in China

Eisenberg has since traveled to China many times studying and observing these energy approaches to medicine. He has seen many remarkable demonstrations and healings. Qi Gong masters have split stones with their hands and foreheads, had trucks driven over them, without bodily harm, and many other sensational acts. In a 1990 *Noetic Sciences Review* article titled, "Energy Medicine in China", Eisenberg states that "more spectacular still is the observation that large numbers of patients said to have biopsy-proven, non-malignant cancer are being treated with ... Qi Gong therapy... Moreover, the Chinese lay press frequently displays headlines such as, "Qi Gong Defeats Breast Cancer.""

On one occasion Dr. Eisenberg witnessed a Qi Gong master plug an electrical wire into a wall socket, and with one hand on this "live" wire and a voltmeter in his other hand, the Qi Gong master "regulated the voltage from 0 to 220 volts, or held the voltage constant, at will, upon my request." Because he was skeptical that this was some kind of high technology trick, he allowed the Qi Gong master to touch him for a split second, long enough to feel the jolt of this electrical current, which would normally cause serious muscle spasm, if not electrocution, when held as long as the Qi Gong master held the wire. Eisenberg reported, "He was 'live' all right." He added:

> In a final demonstration the Qi Gong master took two metal skewers along with a one-pound pork steak, which he had brought with him. He put the two skewers through the steak then grabbed the skewers,

one in the left hand and one in the right so as to complete an electrical circuit. Having grasped the wires along with the two skewers, the circuit was engaged and the pork chop began to smoke and flame. Within minutes there was a medium-well-done pork chop, which my Qi Gong friend sliced and offered to serve! I was astounded by this demonstration and have no adequate explanation for why the Qi Gong master did not injure his skin, or cause a serious heart irregularity, seizure or other damage to his own person.

And while he still is unable to explain scientifically how it is that Qi Gong masters can perform these amazing feats, Dr. Eisenberg is personally convinced of the value and effectiveness of energy medicine treatments.

Acupuncture is the best-known and used traditional Chinese energy medicine in the United States. The World Health Organization endorses acupuncture in the treatment of nearly 40 medical conditions. In 1997 the National Institutes of Health, after reviewing the scientific evidence, recommended integrating acupuncture into standard medical practice, and urged insurance companies to begin paying for acupuncture treatments. They acknowledged the controversial philosophy behind the practice of this ancient therapy, but concluded that acupuncture clearly works to treat a number of medical diagnoses.

Therapeutic Touch

Therapeutic Touch is another well-known and used energy treatment used in the United States. The theory of Therapeutic Touch (TT) is very similar to the earlier mentioned ancient healing practices. In this approach, the practitioner senses or feels the patient's vital energy field, which projects beyond the periphery of the body. When an imbalance is sensed, TT healers move their hands over the "blocked" energy field, much like massage, but without direct body contact. In this focused state of attention, TT healers then modulate the balanced flow of energy with both their thought and the movement of their hands to "unruffle" the person's energy field.

Dr. Dolores Krieger and Dora Kunz developed Therapeutic Touch in 1972. In 1975 Dr. Krieger developed and taught the clinical practice of Therapeutic Touch as part of the Master's Degree Program in Nursing at New York University. Nearly one hundred colleges and universities currently teach TT as an integral part of their nursing programs. Considerable research exists demonstrating its effectiveness, and some can be found in Krieger's 1993 book, *Accepting Your Power to Heal: The Personal Practice of Therapeutic Touch.*

A 2009 study of Therapeutic Touch was conducted at the University of Missouri with patients recovering from surgery. Guy McCormack, who is chair of the Department of Occupational Therapy and Occupational Science in the School of Health Professions, headed this research. Ninety patients were divided into a TT treatment group, placebo group, and a no-treatment control group. The results were that 73% of patients receiving TT had a significant reduction in pain, had fewer requests for medication, and slept more comfortably following surgery. Patients in the other groups reported increased pain. McCormack commented, "Although it is difficult to introduce this form of therapy into medical settings, more and more hospitals are using complementary therapies like TT because consumers are interested in abandoning pharmacological solutions for pain, and instead are interested in harnessing their own capacity to heal through an inexpensive and cost-effective process."

I first observed the effectiveness of Therapeutic Touch when I invited a registered nurse from Penn State's nursing faculty to explain this approach as part of the services I developed for cancer centers. She invited volunteers from the audience to come to the front of the room, where she moved her hands over their bodies, sensing their energy field. In every instance she correctly diagnosed the body part of the patient's disease or illness with no medical records or any other objective data to aid her diagnosis!

In 1995, my wife Shelly, who was then a massage therapist, began to study Therapeutic Touch. In 1996 I joined her at a workshop presented by Dr. Krieger. Since then I have observed my wife's ability to dramatically affect physical symptoms. Two of the examples of my wife's use of TT are with personal friends, both of whom are physicians.

In the summer of 1994 or 1995, we held one of our picnics for cancer patients in State College, Pennsylvania in conjunction with an American Cancer Society event. Somehow I convinced a group of physicians to participate and to sit in a "dunk tank." People at the picnic would throw a ball, and if it hit the target, this released the person, who would fall into the tank full of water. To this day I still can't believe I talked these doctors into doing this. But, of course, the patients loved it.

One of the participants was Dr. Jerry Derdel, who was Medical Director of Radiation Oncology at this hospital. Jerry was one of the last physician volunteers to be dunked. I didn't really pay attention, but as the afternoon wore on, and the doctors kept getting dunked, quite a bit of water had been splashed out of the tank, which we didn't think to refill. Jerry happens to be fairly tall, and in the process of getting dunked, he thought he had broken his toe. He told me that he had to leave to go to the hospital to have his foot x-rayed.

Jerry was familiar with my interest in alternative therapy approaches, but I didn't know how well he'd respond to my suggestion that he let my wife help him. I decided to at least offer Shelly's assistance. Fortunately, Jerry allowed Shelly to practice TT for his injured toe.

The next morning, Jerry told us that x-rays confirmed the broken toe. He was prepared for the worst, including a slow, painful time to heal. To his surprise, however, he said that he had taken no pain medication, went for a long ride on his bicycle, and had no symptoms at all. He admitted his inability to understand what she had done, but was personally convinced that what Shelly had done had made the difference.

On another occasion we were at dinner with Dr. Ted Ziff, Director of Emergency Medicine at this same hospital. During the evening Ted explained that he had pulled a muscle in his back that afternoon while gardening in his yard. When we got back to Ted's house, he could hardly stand upright and clearly was in pain. Shelly convinced Ted to let her use TT on his back.

The next morning Ted called from the hospital to thank Shelly. He had had this type of injury a number of times before, and it had always kept him at home in pain, sometimes for days. Following this type of muscle strain, he had never been able to go to work the next day, but here he was at work feeling better than ever. He conceded that there was nothing medically he could have done to affect himself this way. He was especially pleased and impressed.

Therapeutic Touch is similar to other approaches such as laying-on of hands, faith healing, and spiritual healing. In her book, *Hands of Light: A Guide to Healing Through the Human Energy Field*, Barbara Brennan describes these approaches as procedures that involve re-balancing the human energy field.

As a child Brennan spent considerable time alone in the woods around her home, and realized that:

> In those quiet moments in the woods I entered into an expanded state of consciousness in which I was able to perceive things beyond the normal human ranges of experience. I remember knowing where each small animal was without looking. I could sense its state. When I practiced walking blindfolded in the woods, I would feel the trees long before I could touch them with my hands. I realized that the trees were larger than they appeared to the visible eye. Trees have life energy fields around them, and I was sensing those fields. Later I learned to see the energy fields of trees and the small animals. I discovered

that everything has an energy field around it that looks somewhat like the light from a candle. I also began to notice that everything was connected by these energy fields, that no space existed without an energy field. Everything, including me, was living in a sea of energy.

Brennan says that she "accepted it all as perfectly natural, assumed everyone knew it, and then I forgot about it." It wasn't until later in her life, after completing a masters degree in atmospheric physics and working for NASA doing research, that she says "I began seeing colors around people's heads", which were similar to experiences of her "clairvoyant vision" in childhood. This ultimately led her to discover that she could diagnose and heal people.

She is now a highly regarded spiritual healer and teaches her approach in the Barbara Brennan School of Healing. She says that when one enters an expanded state of consciousness, such as in meditation, you begin to see a greater reality that is beyond the normal human perception range:

If a person is unhealthy, it will show in his energy field as an unbalanced flow of energy and/or stagnated energy that has ceased to flow and appears as darkened colors. In contrast, a healthy person shows bright colors that flow easily in a balanced field. These colors and forms are very specific to each illness.

In the process of learning to see these energy fields or human auras, she also found herself intuitively receiving information about a person's illness and what she and the client could do to rebalance the energy field. Examples of these auras are illustrated in her books *Hands of Light* (1988) and *Light Emerging* (1993).

There is scientific evidence to support the existence of these energy fields. I already mentioned how in 1935 Dr. Harold Saxton Burr developed an "electrodynamic theory of life," and proposed that these "fields of life" (L-fields) are the electronic matrix, which regulates the biological form.

His research measuring the electrical properties of plant seeds showed a significant relationship between the initial measured potential of the seed and the actual growth of the plant. In one study, the electrical fields of corn seeds were measured and placed in high, medium, and low potential groups. When the seeds were planted under controlled conditions in the field, the growth and yield of the seeds correlated with their electrical potential. When the seeds from these plants were replanted, the results were even more striking. When seeds from these second generation plants were measured, they correlated highly again with the original grouping of high, medium, or low potential.

Burr's research also demonstrated that the energy field of an organism in its initial stage determines its future shape or adult form. For example, he found that the shape of the energy field around tiny seedlings resembled the shape of the adult plant. He also determined that abnormal voltage patterns could "give warning of something 'out of shape' in the body," and predict a disease process.

Dr. Louis Langman, from the Department of Obstetrics and Gynecology, New York University College of Medicine, used this technique to predict and confirm uterine cancer in 95 of 102 patients. In another study with 428 patients he determined that the microvolt meter could measure obvious differences in malignant or non-malignant status of the cervix of these women. These studies were aided by grants from the National Cancer Institute.

In the 1940's, Kirlean photography also demonstrated the existence of energy fields. Russian researcher Semyon Kirlean showed that plants, animals, and humans discharge an "electrical corona" from their bodies, which can be measured with electrophotography. He, and many others since, have found that the corona pattern can diagnose disease.

Many of you are likely familiar with the "phantom leaf effect." When a portion of a leaf is cut off and filmed by electrophotography, the developed photograph shows a picture of the whole leaf. Similar research has shown that if you cut a hole in a leaf, the electrophotograph reveals the full leaf with yet another smaller leaf with a hole in it appearing within the hole of the larger leaf. Richard Gerber's research has confirmed this effect, which suggests an "etheric body" or "holographic energy template that guides the growth and development of the physical body." He concluded, "The Phantom Leaf Effect would seem to confirm the holographic nature of the organizing energy field that surrounds all living systems."

Holograms

A hologram is created by splitting a single laser beam in two. When the original laser beam is now directed to interact and reflect light from the split laser light, an interference pattern is created, which can be photographed. When you cut the film of the object into pieces, each piece when now viewed through a pure laser light will display a miniature replica of the whole object.

Holograms demonstrate a fundamental principle in nature: Every cell of a living structure contains the blueprint for the entire organism. This phenomenon is well researched in cellular biology. Every cell in the body contains the genetic material necessary to recreate the entire human body. This is the principle used in cloning research. I discussed this in Chapter 6, and how energy fields affect cell growth and health.

In *Vibrational Medicine*, Gerber speculates further:

> Perhaps the universe itself is a gigantic "cosmic hologram." *That is to say, the universe is a tremendous energy interference pattern.* By virtue of its likely holographic characteristics, every piece of the universe not only contains but also contributes to the information of the whole. The cosmic hologram is less like a holographic still photo frozen in time than it is like a holographic videotape dynamically changing from moment to moment.

A January 15, 2009 article titled "Our world may be a giant hologram" in *New Scientist* by Marcus Chown has given decided support to the possibility that we are living in a cosmic hologram. Dr. Craig Hogan is Director of

Fermilab's Center for Particle Astrophysics in Batavia, Illinois. He has been part of the GEO600 laser experiment for the past seven years, and has been attempting to detect gravitational waves from "super-dense astronomical objects such as neutron stars and black holes." Hogan believes:

> GEO600 has stumbled upon the fundamental limit of space-time – the point where space-time stops behaving like the smooth continuum Einstein described and instead dissolves into 'grains,' just as a newspaper photograph dissolves into dots as you zoom in… At this magnification, the fabric of space-time becomes grainy and is ultimately made of tiny units rather like pixels, but a hundred billion billion times smaller than a proton.

While more research needs to be done, Hogan suggests, "We may have our first indication of how space-time emerges out of quantum theory." This holographic principle could help describe what is happening at the most fundamental level of the universe. This has been a major premise of physicist Dr. David Bohm.

Bohm wrote and taught extensively that separateness is an illusion, and that the universe is like a hologram. Just as any piece of the hologram is the image of the entire hologram, Bohm proposed that any information about the universe or "all that is" is contained in any part. He called this underlying matrix of oneness the "implicate order", which is "enfolded" into the universe. We see only what is in the "explicate order" based on our physical senses. It's all vibration or "wave forms." Our physical senses can sense or detect only a very small range of these frequencies.

I want to give you a sense of just how little we know about our explicate or physical reality. Sounds are frequencies vibrating between 0 and 20,000 cycles per second. Colors are frequencies vibrating between approximately 400 to nearly 800 billion cycles per second. The difference between the colors red and orange and yellow, etc. is the speed that the wave is vibrating. We have senses that vibrate in harmony with these ranges of frequencies and are able to sense them as hearing and sight. If you took all of the frequency ranges that we are able to sense with our physical senses and compared them to all of the known physical ranges, including what can be detected with X-rays, it would be less than one inch compared to a mile. Based on what we can measure scientifically, I hope you can see that we know extremely little about our universe or reality.

You can read about Bohm's theories in his 1980 book, *Wholeness and the Implicate Order*. A primary tenet of his theory of what he calls the "holoverse" is that all of reality is a dynamic process. Remember the idea that something only takes form when we're observing or measuring it. "In a holographic universe, even time and space could no longer be viewed as fundamentals. Because concepts such as location break down in a universe in which nothing is truly separate from anything else." The ultimate nature of reality is an undivided whole in perpetual flux, what he calls "holomovement." He adds that above and beyond the implicate order is a superimplicate order and maybe a whole hierarchy of implicate orders. This superimplicate order is analogous to archetypes or Sheldrake's morphogenetic fields.

Sheldrake and Bohm believe that there is an overlap between science and metaphysics, where only compassion and order are possible in the implicate order. Rene Weber discusses this in Ken Wilber's book, *The Holographic Paradigm*. There is a "beyond" that is beyond the explicate and implicate. There is an ultimate source of all. We call this the sacred, spirit, holy, transcendent, God – it just is. We can reach this Divine Consciousness through meditation or related altered states of consciousness, but it cannot be measured or grasped through thought. Bohm openly dialogued with the Indian spiritual master and mystic, J. Krishnamurti, and the Dalai Lama, where they discussed the existence of pure awareness beyond thought. Bohm's superimplicate order could be conceptualized as the source of spiritual knowledge and wisdom. His research suggests, "Physics can be rigorously consistent with the existence of higher realms of truth, order, existence, and eternity."

That quantum physics appears to be saying much of what ancient religions and mystics have espoused comes from several sources. This was presented well in *The Tao of Physics* by Fritjof Capra and in *The Dancing WuLi Masters* by Gary Zukav. They noted clear parallels with Taoism, Buddhism, and Hinduism. Dossey similarly states in *Recovering The Soul* "that reasons can still be given *within* science for the existence of the soul and its affinity with God."

In *The Field* and her review of quantum physics, McTaggart believes that the evidence offers a scientific explanation for many ancient mystical and religious beliefs. She suggests that the Chinese belief in the life force energy Qi, and what Christians term the Holy Spirit, is highly related to the quantum field. It even echoes "the Old Testament's account of God's first dictum, 'Let there be light,' out of which matter was created."

McTaggart notes that the pioneers of quantum physics (Erwin Schrödinger, Werner Heisenberg, Niels Bohr, and Wolfgang Pauli) realized the metaphysical correlations of their research and conclusions. If electrons are connected everywhere at once, this suggests the oneness of the universe that is a belief of all major philosophies and religions. These eminent scientists studied classical philosophical texts in order to help them understand their observations. They were aware that their research dramatically challenged the existing laws of physics. McTaggart believes that, "They offered us, in a sense, a science of religion." And today, scientists from the world's finest universities continue to provide "scientific validation of areas which have largely been the domain of religion, mysticism, alternative medicine or New Age speculation."

Norman Shealy

Dr. Norm Shealy is one of these leading researchers and practitioners. He is best known for his innovative approaches to pain management, and for founding the American Holistic Medical Association in 1978. He served as president of the International Society for the Study of Subtle Energies and Energy Medicine, and is Professor of Energy Medicine at Holos University, where with Dr. Caroline Myss, the first doctoral program in energy medicine began in 2001.

Like Larry Dossey, he has been highly instrumental in educating and promoting the need to include spirituality within health care. In fact, he and Dr. Dawson Church state in their book, *Soul Medicine*, "that paying attention to your spiritual life is the most important thing you can do for your health". Their twelve characteristics common to people with a vibrant soul connection include: 1) forgiveness, 2) tolerance, 3) serenity, 4) faith, 5) reason, 6) hope, 7) motivation, 8) consistency, 9) community, 10) joy, 11) gratitude, and 12) love.

The premise of this 2006 book is that good health requires that human consciousness reflects and transmits a connection with one's soul. Health and healing flow through this soul connection, and soul medicine's approach is to facilitate the free expression of the soul in the patient's energy system. Their following quote is in perfect agreement with why I believe love heals:

> When we consciously bring our minds and hearts to a similar vibration, so that they are functioning in the same vibrational range as our soul, then there is resonance between them, and reciprocal communication between their energies. This allows healing to flow effortlessly through to the body.

They also note the need for a resonance between the practitioner and the patient. It has been demonstrated that a healer with a strong healing intention can literally entrain patients' bodily systems to resonate with the healer, leading to a healing response. This is yet another demonstration why love heals. I have experienced this personally in my training and practice of PSYCH-K, a program developed by psychotherapist, Rob Williams.

I was actually attending a PSYCH-K training workshop one weekend when a suicidal patient of mine called for help. Using a process I had learned in this workshop, I was able to send a healing intention that I am certain had a remarkable transforming effect on this woman's emotional state. Because of my interest in guided imagery I have been aware of this phenomenon for some time. Jeanne Achterberg and her book, *Imagery in Healing: Shamanism and Modern Medicine*, have been a valuable resource for me in understanding the power of healing intention throughout history.

Shealy and Church also note an unusual spiritual phenomenon: the incorruptible bodies of saints. One of my best friends, James Barrett, explores this also in his book, *The Silent Gospel*. In the third chapter of his book, James reports that several spiritual figures, who when they died, their bodies remained free of decay for extensive time periods – years, even decades. This has been well documented. The explanation for the attainment of this "rainbow body" is that certain yoga practitioners and "true saints" are able to rearrange their vibratory structure.

Pure Consciousness

I'd like to add a personal soul-connection story. I was invited to speak at the Academy for Guided Imagery's annual conference in November 2000, co-sponsored with the Biofeedback Society of California. Another presenter was a Japanese yoga master, Mitsumasa Kawakami. As part of his lunchtime presentation, Mr. Kawakami demonstrated remarkable ability to control his body. At first he literally skewered his tongue and neck with long needles, without any apparent pain, bleeding, or evidence that they had been punctured.

Following this he held up a double-edged knife, and showed how very sharp it was. Then he asked for two volunteers to join him on stage to squeeze his hand around this knife. He asked for another volunteer to come and pull the knife through his hand while the two others were applying full pressure. I was the volunteer who pulled the knife through his hand.

The most amazing thing happened – I don't know when I started or when I stopped pulling the knife. There was no resistance whatsoever. At some point I simply realized that I was holding the knife. I had been very concerned that I would do something that would cut his hand severely. Yet his hand was completely unharmed. I was stunned. I asked Mr. Kawakami how he was able to do this: What was going on in his mind when we were squeezing and pulling? Through a Japanese interpreter he responded, "I was one with the knife. The knife and I are made of the same fundamental stuff. I trusted that in my sense of being one with the knife, it would not cut me."

I was both surprised and not surprised by what he said. It actually made sense to me theoretically. The thing that got me was that he had actually applied this understanding of oneness! He clearly demonstrated that humans have this ability to transcend the physical. As he explains in a pamphlet, *The Essence of the Kawakami School of Yoga*, the purpose of his school is to teach how "to move one's thoughts and actions to a higher and more pure plane."

Following the lunch and presentation, Mr. Kawakami and his entourage approached me, and expressed what I thought was unusual interest in me and my book, *Doctor's Orders: Go Fishing*, which was newly released at the time. We had never met before, and they had no prior knowledge of my work or me. Except, it turns out they did.

Shortly after this conference I received a phone call from the Japanese interpreter. They wanted to meet and speak with me. I was confused since I don't speak Japanese, and wasn't sure about the purpose of our getting together. She explained that at a soul level they "knew" they had to meet me. I was certainly surprised by her answer. Further, I assumed I would travel to San Francisco, where the interpreter lived, thinking that Mr. Kawakami would have another reason to return there from Japan. In fact, their only reason to return to the States was to meet me!

Now, I'm a practical kind of guy. I couldn't help but think to myself that this was a bit much. Just think of the time and expense alone for them to fly from Japan just to meet me. Of course, I readily accepted, and invited their group to stay at our home. In April 2001, Mr. Kawakami's Principle Director of his Tokyo Ashram, Misa Sata, and two student assistants, and the interpreter, Yuko Franklin, visited for a 3-day weekend. Mr. Kawakami did not attend (part of Japanese tradition), but did come to visit in July with Misa, a student assistant (Tomoko), and Yuko. They made a second trip from Japan solely to visit for another weekend!

They were glad to have this opportunity to tell me about their work at the Kawakami School of Yoga and the Institute for Research of Subconscious Psychology. And they were sincerely interested in my work and research. But, of course, this went deeper. Misa and Mr. Kawakami claimed that they knew me from prior lifetimes where we similarly pioneered new approaches to health. Mr. Kawakami also reflected fondly on our relationship when I was his younger brother. Their souls genuinely wanted to reconnect with my wife and me, although I have to admit I had no conscious sense of this connection.

But now I'd like to add to the above story. In March 2002 Mr. Kawakami was invited to give a special presentation to the annual meeting of the Association for Applied Psychophysiology and Biofeedback in Las Vegas. Dr. Erik Peper, a biofeedback expert and Professor in the Department of Health Education at San Francisco State University, co-presented with Mr. Kawakami. Essentially, they had wired Mr. Kawakami to every known monitoring device, so that they could record (and the audience could see) his ability to control pain and bleeding when he pierced his tongue and neck with a 2-millimeter needle.

I had been invited to give a full-day workshop in Las Vegas to the Nevada Occupational Therapist's Association, and, fortunately, was able to schedule this the same time Mr. Kawakami was in town. While I knew how well he could affect bodily control and healing, I have to admit that it still amazed me to see him do it. But, what was extra interesting this time, I found myself standing next to Dr. Beverly Rubik.

I had met Beverly at a holistic health conference where we were both presenters at Penn State University. I mentioned her earlier related to her expertise in subtle energies. She is a biophysicist and served as a member of the advisory panel to the National Institutes of Health office of Alternative Medicine, and was panel chair on Bioelectromagnetics. So, I was taken by Beverly's reaction to Mr. Kawakami. As experienced as she was with subtle energies and having been Director of the Center for Frontier Sciences at Temple University for many years, even Beverly was amazed at his demonstration. She kept shaking her head and saying that he shows no indication of any trauma reaction in his body on any of the physiological recordings. None.

The next day Mr. Kawakami was gracious enough to join me at my presentation for the occupational therapists. They, too, were awed by what the mind can do. Once again, Mr. Kawakami demonstrated and explained that he simply communicated with the needle while he entered a deep state of concentration and meditation. He claims that this "union of one's soul with purest consciousness" can lead to "self-liberation" or "release from all restraints to find complete freedom for the body, mind and soul." The key is recognizing the existence of your soul, and connecting your soul or pure spirit with the cosmic truth of oneness and universal love.

Chapter 9 - Intuition

Another component of Dossey's Era III medicine and Shealy's soul medicine is the use of one's intuition. Both offer considerable compelling evidence, including significant research, validating "psychic functioning." It is remarkable to me that so much literature exists supporting intuition and psychic phenomena, and, still, some doubt the evidence. I actually devoted two chapters in *Doctor's Orders: Go Fishing* to intuition because I had extensive experience with it personally, as well as teaching it in my classes and many workshops.

Intuition by definition is knowledge based on insight or spiritual perception rather than on reasoning. It's entirely subjective. On the surface, it's the antithesis of objective science. However, I'd like to demonstrate to you that we use or experience intuition all the time.

For example, most women would admit to having and using their intuition as a natural part of who they are. Men, though, tend to treat this as a feminine trait to be tolerated, but not often respected. Interestingly, however, it is not uncommon for men to talk about their gut feelings. But aren't gut feelings really a form of intuition?

For years I attended weekly cancer conferences or "tumor boards" where physicians presented specific medical cases in order to discuss treatment options for their cancer patients. It was not considered inappropriate for doctors to offer their clinical experience, "impressions," or gut feelings in these discussions. In fact, if you think about it, wouldn't it be quite helpful to have a group of experts share their clinical experience and gut feelings? Wouldn't you be glad to have this additional insight?

Another intriguing question is, would you be open to a doctor's insights and guidance that came through prayer or some spiritual means? Is it unreasonable to think that healthcare professionals could or would have spiritual assistance? In his book, *Reinventing Medicine*, Dossey notes, "the path of the physician since antiquity has been considered a spiritual path and remains so." He believes that most physicians have an "intrinsic sensitivity to spiritual issues," but that this is challenging because it is so foreign to their medical training, which focuses on the mechanical, objective, and rational.

Dossey encourages physicians to consider a website created by psychologist and Professor Emeritus, Charles Tart, of the University of California at Davis. This website (www.issc-taste.org) called The Archives of Scientists' Transcendent Experiences (TASTE), states that "it is an online journal devoted to transcendent experiences that scientists have reported. It lets scientists express these experiences in a safe space, collects and shares them to debunk the stereotype that 'real' scientists don't have 'spiritual' or 'mystical' or 'psychic' experiences, builds a database of these experiences for future research, and helps us understand the full range of human mind." I strongly recommend anyone to read these very personal transcendent experiences as reported by hundreds of objectively trained scientists.

The fact is, prayer is an important part of the daily life of about 75% of Americans. We think that it's highly appropriate to consult any number of professionals regarding our health or any other matter. Why wouldn't we also choose to consult God or some other spiritual figure or divine resource?

Currently, approximately two-thirds of Americans report having experienced extra sensory perception (ESP). Nearly one-half of American adults believe that they have been in contact with someone who has died, usually a dead spouse or sibling. About one-half of Americans believe that their pet dogs respond to their thoughts. And even the U.S. Central Intelligence Agency (CIA) admitted publicly in 1995 to conducting more than 20 years of research using intuition as a means of intelligence collection.

Almost all artists, writers, composers, and inventors have used intuition in their creative artistic expression. Pitirim Sorokin states in his best-selling book, *The Crisis of Our Age*, "there is hardly any doubt that intuition is the real source of knowledge, different from the role of the senses and reason." His survey of the literature found that philosophers including Plato, Aristotle, Plotinus, St. Augustine, Descartes, Thomas Hobbs, Henri Bergson, Baruch Spinoza, Carl Jung, and Alfred North Whitehead all agreed that intuition is the basis of truth.

Yet another consideration of intuition is from a quantum physics perspective. In her book, *The Field*, Lynn McTaggart discusses research and conversations with Bernie Haisch, an astrophysicist at Lockheed, and Hal Puthoff, a laser physicist. They were instrumental in determining that all matter is really energy, and have used this knowledge to create anti-gravity space travel. They reasoned that the quantum or zero point field, which connected and contained the universe, "had imprinted everything that ever happened in the world through wave interference encoding," and acted like a non-biochemical "memory" in the universe. McTaggart states:

> The Field demonstrated that the real currency of the universe – the very reason for its stability – is an exchange of energy. If we were all connected through The Field, then it just might be possible to tap into this vast reservoir of energy information and extract information from it.

Remember the research where two split protons communicated faster than the speed of light. This suggests the oneness or connectedness of everything. The reason these protons could respond instantaneously to each other is because of their quantum connection. There is no "here" or "there" at the quantum level. The split protons never left from anywhere, nor had to travel anywhere. I'd like to use this information and the law of sympathetic resonance to explain how intuition could work scientifically.

A practical way to describe this would be with the example of a tuning fork. In tuning a piano, the tuner strikes a tuning fork and adjusts the string of each piano key so that it is the same frequency as the tuning fork. Now imagine that there were a room full of tuning forks, all freely suspended (that is, none of them were lying against another surface – they're all hanging from the ceiling separately). When the tuner strikes a tuning fork, it will vibrate and hum. And if one of the other freely suspended tuning forks is the same frequency, it will also vibrate and hum. Literally, when you strike the tuning fork, its movement sends out a frequency, which will cause another tuning fork to vibrate if it is the same frequency (or harmonic).

Since everything is energy, and energy can never be destroyed (only change form), every thought that has ever been thought remains as energy somewhere (or everywhere) in space. In theory, then, one could get information on any subject that has ever been thought, simply by desiring that information. The law of sympathetic resonance would naturally attract or communicate with something on the same frequency or thought. Thus, when praying, meditating, or dreaming, you could ask for and receive (intuit) information on whatever you want.

Divine Revelation, Dreams, and Prophecy

The fact is that every culture in recorded history has used divine revelation and dreams for spiritual guidance. Many of the world's religions have their origins in dreams. The Arabic prophet, Muhammad, was given spiritual insights by the angel Gabriel. Most of this guidance in founding the religion of Muhammadanism and the content of the Koran was revealed to him through his dreams. Joseph Smith was ordained a prophet based on revelation from an angel, which became the Book of Mormon and the foundation for the church of Jesus Christ of Latter-Day Saints in 1830. The Buddha's birth was announced to his mother, Queen Maza, in a dream, where it was foretold that he would become a spiritual leader. The birth of Jesus was similarly announced to his mother, Mary. And the Emperor Constantine declared Christianity the official religion of the Roman Empire when he dreamed of marking a Christian symbol on the shields of his soldiers to use as a safeguard in battle.

In his book, *Dreams: The Dark Speech of the Spirit*, Morton Kelsey reports:

> No hard and fast lines were drawn between the state of dreaming as we understand it and the state of trance of the ecstatic consciousness in which a vision was received. Sometimes two or three quite different names were used to speak of a single experience, and at times it is difficult to be sure which state was signified by the writer. All of them – dream, vision, and trance – were valued to such a degree that there was no urgent need to distinguish one another.

This was the basic attitude shared by Christianity, Judaism, and the Hellenistic world.

Dreams remained an important tool for the early Christian community. In the fifth century, Augustine, Sunesius, Ambrose and others wrote clearly supporting the use of dreams. But the Roman Empire had fallen, and education and culture had declined. The dark ages were beginning.

Two highly influential church leaders at this time were Jerome and Gregory. Both valued dreams and visions, but also saw them as potential for demonic influence. Dreams then became associated with witchcraft, soothsaying, and related superstitious ideas. Morton Kelsey reports that the growing ignorance and superstition of a dying culture now began to lead the Christian church to ignore the value of dreams.

Things changed drastically in the Middle Ages. While the early Greeks, Hebrews, and Christians revered dreams as a vehicle for communication from the Divine, the medieval church feared any questioning of its authority. Confidence in a direct contact with God through dreams was just such a threat. Kelsey suggests, "all necessary truth about God had been laid down and men didn't need direct contact with him anymore."

The fact is that psychic phenomena have always been a part of religion. Ancestor worship (conversing with the dead) has been common practice. Many historians believe that religion was born out of a need to answer paranormal phenomena such as apparitions and related after-life occurrences. In fact, apparitions may be the seed of all theology. When people were seen as an apparition after they had died, the concept of being saved developed. The belief that the gods spared this person opened the way to heaven and a way to conquer death for all believers.

As noted earlier, ancient wisdom proposes that life's purpose is realizing the enduring connection to a greater whole, or oneness with God. Humans throughout history knew of this connection through personal mystical, peak, or transcendent experiences. This included mediumship or trance communication with the gods. This deep sense of the belonging of the individual to Spirit has been told by prophets throughout the ages.

Early evidence of gods speaking through prophets is seen in the famous oracles in Greece and the Near East at least eleven centuries B.C. The word "oracle" meant the place where a deity might be consulted, but it also became used for the god who gave the answer or for the reply itself. This is reported in the acclaimed book, *With the Tongues of Men and Angels*. "The oracles were essential for cities, tribes, and individuals to provide authority and advice in conducting affairs of state, religious matters, and everyday lives." Perhaps the best known is the oracle of Apollo at Delphi in Greece where the famous inscription "Know Thyself" was written on the temple.

It was common for these prophets to speak while in a trance state. The Biblical prophets, Jeremiah, Isaiah, and Micah, often communicated their messages through trance. In medieval Jewish practice many rabbis had a maggid, a spiritual teacher who spoke to and through them. The Hebrew prophets claimed to speak the words of Yahweh. And, as I noted earlier, the Arabic prophet, Muhammad, spoke the words of the angel, Gabriel.

Until the invention of the printing press in 1450, people relied on priests, monks, and orthodoxy for their knowledge. Prior to this, no one in the general populous could read or write. In fact, it wasn't until Martin Luther was excommunicated from the Roman Catholic Church in the sixteen century that the Bible came into prominence. Luther needed a divine authority, and he turned to the newly printed Bible, which came to be known as the "paper Pope."

Science and Other Evidence

The 14th to the 16th centuries were the Renaissance period of thought and reason, and initiated the use of the scientific method to determine truth. History is very clear that religions and governments often used this time of ignorance as a way to control their people. But now religious beliefs, which are the realm of faith, were going to be challenged by objectively measured fact. And as the nature of the universe and the physical body came to be viewed as mechanistic, spiritual questions such as life having meaning and purpose, and the use of intuition and spiritual guidance, came under scientific scrutiny.

In the seventeenth century Sir Isaac Newton determined that natural, not supernatural, law ran the universe. In the nineteenth century Charles Darwin championed the role of evolution over spiritual creation of the universe. Thought, reason, and science now dominated the use of intuition as the way to determine truth.

Interestingly, while science was establishing its foothold, psychical research was one of the major fields of investigation at the end of the nineteenth century. William James, a Harvard professor and physician and one of the world's most highly regarded intellects, was one of the pioneers in researching paranormal events such as telepathy, mediumship, mental healing, and survival after death. He established the first psychology research laboratory at Harvard University, and is considered the father of experimental psychology. He was a long-standing member of the British Society for Psychical Research, and served as its president in 1894 and 1895.

The book, *William James on Psychical Research*, clearly states that he was fully convinced of the ability of some "mediums" to have "supernormal knowledge... Knowledge that cannot be traced to the ordinary sources of information..." This book was the compilation of William James' research in psychical phenomena, and was edited by Gardner Murphy who was then Director of Research at the Menninger Foundation.

Dr. Murphy was President of the American Psychological Association in 1944, and author of many books on psychology and parapsychology, including *Challenge of Psychical Research*. Gardner Murphy, like William James, was strongly aware of the fraud and lack of scientific proof for much of the claims in this field, but he, like James, was convinced of the considerable "serious evidence... of psychical happenings."

A notable example of the use of intuition in this century is the *Course in Miracles*, a text that was dictated over seven years to a highly unlikely recipient, a Professor of Medical Psychology at Columbia University's College of Physicians and Surgeons. In 1965, Dr. Helen Schucman began to have highly symbolic dreams, strange images, and heard an "inner voice", which said, "This is a course in miracles. Please take notes."

Dr. Schucman took the "inner dictation" in shorthand, and her colleague, Dr. William Thetford, supported her and typed the complete manuscript of 1500 pages. Both Schucman and Thetford were anything but religious, but decided to record the information that was decidedly Christian and spiritual. The text was published in 1975, and currently millions of people ascribe to the fundamental principle of the book: how to obtain inner peace.

An excellent summary about *A Course in Miracles* and a survey of the study of "channeling" or "mediums" can be found in the book, *With the Tongues of Men and Angels: A Study of Channeling,* by Arthur Hastings. In the preface to the book he concludes "that there are exceptional levels of creativity and wisdom that are accessible to us, regardless of where we believe they originate."

What is currently called channeling has existed since the beginning of recorded human history. The process is one in which information, ideas, creative works, and personal guidance come to our minds from a source outside our own selves. The individual's mind seems to act as a receiver for another communicator. This book uses the term channeling because it is current, but the process has been called prophecy, oracle, revelation, spirit communication, possession, and the inspiration of the muses. The biblical tradition on Judaism and Christianity says that the prophets received and spoke the words of God. Today, there are many individuals who speak words that are said to come from disembodied teachers on other levels of reality. The process, though not necessarily the content, appears to be the same.

A recent example of this kind of spiritual insight being given in a seemingly unlikely scenario was in 1992 when Neale Donald Walsch began to write about his conversations with God. He had a years-long habit of writing about his thoughts and feelings when one day, after writing a letter to God, his pen began "moving on its own." He said that the experience was not so much like writing, but like "taking dictation." Six years later he had completed these conversations and published them in three books, *Conversations With God: Book One, Two*, and *Three*.

Walsch found himself asking questions that were very personal to him, like: "How does God talk, and to whom?" And to his great surprise he was given the answer in *Book One*, "I talk to everyone. All the time. The question is not to whom do I talk, but who listens?"

Conversations With God: Book 1, first published in 1995, remained on the New York Times bestseller list through 1999. All three books have been read by millions of people. And I am especially pleased to say that I, personally, have been very moved by the wisdom presented in these books. And, also in the books by Esther and Jerry Hicks, where Esther channels a spiritual consciousness named Abraham.

Caroline Myss

Another outstanding example of the use of intuition in recent history is the work of Dr. Caroline Myss, a "medical intuitive." Myss has the unique ability to diagnose people's medical condition without ever having had any formal medical training. She reports that her ability to intuit people's illness was "a type of curiosity" that she normally participated in at her leisure. She was originally trained as a journalist and became a book publisher. But in 1984 she met Dr. Norman Shealy, who had a personal interest in intuitive diagnosis. Dr. Shealy asked Myss if she would be willing to be "tested" and to work with him clinically to diagnose and help his patients. The arrangement was for Dr. Shealy to telephone Myss from his office 1200 miles away, and give her the patient's name and birth date. Myss would then give her "impressions" of the person's medical condition.

Most of the information that Myss intuitively received and reported to Shealy regarded patients' personality conflicts and the impact of their heartache, grief, rage, or love on their physical body. She claims that this emotional, psychological, and spiritual stress is the cause of and "indicator as to what physical dysfunctions exist in the patient's body."

Many Eastern traditions, such as the practice of acupuncture, emphasize the human being as a system of energy. Myss says that she can sense this flow of energy through the body, and that where it is blocked indicates what organs and bodily functions are diseased or dysfunctional, and also, what the underlying emotional and psychological stresses are.

Over a three-year period of testing Myss's ability to diagnose several hundred of his patients, Shealy claims that she was 93% accurate. In 1988 they co-authored a book, *The Creation of Health*, where they discuss their work, and what they believe are the underlying emotional, psychological, and spiritual factors that affect health and healing. In the second part of this book, Shealy explains the medical reasons for developing a particular illness, and Myss follows with the "energy" factor.

She generally believes that what makes people ill is "a strong dose of negativity and fear." Myss states:

> Specifically, we all need to love and to be loved. When love is missing from our lives, our health diminishes. We all need to have something that gives our lives

meaning. Without meaning, our health
slowly, but most certainly, evaporates.

One of the diseases they discuss is
Temporomandibular Joint Syndrome or TMJ. Dr. Shealy
reports, "It occurs because of chronic severe muscle
tension in the jaw muscles with grinding of the teeth and
irritation of the joint that we use in speaking and in
chewing." Carolyn Myss follows with her energy analysis
of TMJ:

> The causes of stress in the jaw
> muscles are multiple, though they all stem
> from tension resulting from blockages
> concerning the use of one's will power and
> self-expression.
> One source of this stress is the
> inability to articulate verbally what one
> needs to say. Whether this block is caused
> by a fear of rejection, criticism or insecurity
> rooted in the fear of losing one's physical
> base of security, the experience of physical
> tension and teeth-grinding is the same.
> Another source of this stress is that
> the grinding of teeth, like fingernail-biting
> or gum-chewing, becomes a habit one does
> unconsciously as a release of tension. Yet
> another source is that the jaw area becomes
> the receptacle for the energies of anger and
> frustration, holding the "words" one would
> like to say to someone but cannot, for
> whatever reasons.

Any time a person's power of choice, personal development in terms of self-expression, or creative expression is stifled, there is negative residue and this can lodge in the jaw as well. This dysfunction is remarkably common because the issues that create it are remarkably common.

When I first read *The Creation of Health* and came to this description of TMJ, I was particularly interested because my wife has this condition. I asked her if she would be willing to read Myss's analysis and tell me what she thought. After reading the analysis my wife replied, "It fits me perfectly."

I was very curious about my wife's response, not only because it supported Myss's position, but also because it occurred to me that I might be contributing to my wife's condition. I generally don't have a problem expressing myself, and I decided to talk with my wife about how I might help her with her ability to speak up for herself.

We talked for about twenty minutes and I agreed to be more aware of over-asserting myself, and to be more supportive of her self-expression. The next morning my wife said that it was the first time in years that she did not awake with her TMJ pain. And to this date, whenever she experiences the TMJ, she knows that it's related to her not speaking up for herself. She then addresses the issue, resulting in a lessening or elimination of the jaw pain.

Carolyn Myss has since authored numbers of books and is one of the most popular and successful writers and speakers in the mind-body-spirit field today. All of her books have been *New York Times* best sellers.

Norm Shealy became known because of his effective use of alternative healing techniques in pain management at the Shealy Institute, which he founded in 1971. Much more recently, he and Caroline Myss founded the world's first doctorate program in energy medicine. As part of the curriculum, students are trained to become medically intuitive.

However, Dr. Shealy's primary experience in researching medical intuitives is very interesting. Most of the people he has tested are less than ten percent accurate ninety-nine percent of the time. He states very clearly that good medical intuitives are very, very rare. He's found that even reputable medical intuitives are seldom accurate enough to be of practical use.

This conforms with my colleague, Ken McCaulley's experience. In the 1960's-70's Ken had a personal interest in intuition, interviewed hundreds of "psychics", and attended more than one thousand séances. His conclusion was that most of these people were deluded or dishonest. But what fascinated him was to find that about fifteen percent had a clear ability to discern the truth of something without objective evidence.

As I noted earlier, citing William James' and Gardner Murphy's research and experience, clearly there are people who have exceptional intuitive abilities. But it is important for me to state here that the seeking of serious advice from a so-called medical intuitive can be very risky business.

While Norm Shealy and Ken McCaulley found the great majority of so-called "intuitives" or "psychics" to be inaccurate, what Ken found was that the best and valid "intuitives" were not public about their abilities. They had no need to seek attention for their intuitive gifts.

Ken concluded that intuition is a natural human function. Everyone has this "sixth sense", as we're finding now in studies with humans, animals and plants. Some intuitives are clearly much better than others, and the very best are a distinct minority. But he also was certain that one's intuitive abilities could be developed, which he found to be very true in his own life and with the thousands of people he taught in his classes.

You can learn to discern the truth for yourself. The key is discernment. In time, with practice, you can become quite accurate at knowing what is right for you. It will feel right. And even if what felt right at the time turns out to be less than completely true, my opinion is that it was the right thing for you to do then. It was what you were open to and ready for at that time.

I call it tuning into the "Wisdom Channel". Intuition is a vibration broadcast from your soul or Divine Source. Think of it like tuning into a radio station. The radio wave is there; you just need a receiver, tuner, and amplifier. You just need to be open. In fact, it's all about your openness and intention. God's voice is always with you; you just have to tune in.

It is beyond the scope of this book to chronicle all of the positive findings supporting psychic phenomena and intuitive abilities. Serious inquiries into the subject are included in many books and journals. I especially recommend the research by Dr. Marilyn Schlitz, and Dr. Dean Radin, research scientists for the Institute of Noetic Sciences.

My Personal Experience

I already explained in Chapter 1 how I became interested in parapsychology, including reading the books by Jane Roberts, who was a psychic and trance medium, and channeled a spiritual personality named Seth. Eventually I met Ken McCaulley, and my life was forever changed when for seven years I was able to speak daily to "mentors" and "Master Teachers" who were channeled through Ken. For up to one hour every day for seven years, I spoke with these people from a spiritual dimension who claimed to be assigned to support our decisions and interests and to help us fulfill our life plan. This was all still quite new to me at the time, and a revelation to say the least. Until I met Ken in 1977 at age 33, I had relatively little or no interest in a spiritual life. Still, at that time I was curious and fascinated by all of this, and couldn't really explain why. I now know that it was part of my "soul print" and life plan.

I also noted in Chapter 1 how Ken and I would meditate and practice developing our intuition daily. I was surprised to find that I could use my own intuition and dreams for personal insights. But I surely missed those daily conversations with Ken and our mentors when Ken's health deteriorated rapidly due to a series of strokes in 1985. My interest in intuition continued as I practiced on my own, began my work with Carl Simonton, and taught his "inner guide" approach in my classes and workshops.

I also greatly valued my training with Dr. Martin Rossman and Dr. David Bressler, who were the founders of the Academy for Guided Imagery. They developed a process called interactive guided imagery, where you can gain an enhanced awareness of the unconscious in order to receive insight into any concern. Marty is a general practice physician, and authored the book, *Healing Yourself: A Step-by-Step Program for Better Health Through Imagery*, which I used and recommended most in my clinical practice. He believes that healing is an unconscious process, and has found that you can invite an image of your symptom or problem to come into your conscious awareness, which can reveal information regarding the healing or resolution of the symptom or problem. David is a psychologist and authored the books, *Free Yourself From Pain* and *Health: Toward an Integral Medicine*. He also is founder and former director of the UCLA Pain Control Unit. He similarly used interactive imagery to help people manage chronic pain. You can simply ask your pain to take some form or image, and ask it what you can do to make the pain go away. For those who may be interested, I devote a whole chapter to the "Uses of Intuition in Medicine" in *Doctor's Orders: Go Fishing*.

But 1998 was to be another major turning point. That year my wife and I attended an "Intuition" Conference headed by Larry Dossey, Joan Borysenko, Raymond Moody, Dannion Brinkley, and others. While we thoroughly enjoyed hearing and talking with these recognized authorities about their experience and knowledge regarding intuition, another special treat was meeting Patti Aubrey-Carpenter, a Spiritualist Minister from Cassadega, Florida. She also was a presenter for the conference. Patti's session largely involved her giving "messages" to people in the audience.

During her presentation, Patti told me that I would write a book, among a number of other things that have come true. She also later told Shelly that she was very intuitive, and I was thrilled when Shelly expressed interest in developing her intuition. Once we got home, Shelly immediately was able to access her own inner guide, who called himself "John". So, for the last ten years we have had weekly or monthly conversations with John, who has been an invaluable friend and guide.

The guide, John, along with Ken's and my mentors, have encouraged me to develop my own intuition and not rely on them. At one point they told me that if they gave me the answers to all of my questions (and I had plenty!) all that would prove is that I follow directions well. But the more I learned about their wisdom and the accuracy of their information, I figured I would have been crazy not to ask. However, it was necessary for me, and everyone, to make our own decisions, and that Spirit would support us.

So, my life has been quite an adventure and revelation. I have been blessed in many ways. But nothing compares to my insights gained related to a spiritual side of life and my unending interest to discover Truth. I wrote earlier that Ken was a genuine seeker of Truth and a great friend and mentor. I thought I'd share a poem he wrote titled "dean":

> i looked up.
> there he was!
> i saw him from another time
> when he was garbed in
> gray,
> cowled, searching for a way.
>
> but, here he was,
> bearded again,

light of frame,
penetrating gaze of fire,
almost demanding the riddle
be solved.

dean!

that is what he answers to,
but he answered another time to
warmth,
a smile,
a touch,
years of toil,
denial...
and more.

this time, how is he different?
more accepting, perhaps.
more attuned to cosmos' purpose,
fears allayed,
but still
loving
and always
the friend.

thank god.

dean!

I've added this poem for an extra special reason. Ken died March 15th 1999. I last saw him when he was a patient in a Veteran's Hospital in Michigan before Shelly and I moved to California in 1998. So, you'd think that was the end of my contact with him. Think again.

Sharon Bauer, Ken, David, and another John

A metaphysical shop and bookstore opened last year in the city where I live. I was glad that the owner carried my book in her store, and she asked if I would do a book signing to help promote the book and her store. I was glad to help. There was another author there, too, along with a psychic named Sharon Bauer to give intuitive readings. Business was slow so it gave us lots of time to talk among ourselves.

Sharon confided that she was a good psychic reader, but that she couldn't get intuitive information for herself. I was certain that she could read for herself; it's just that something was blocking her ability to do that. So, we agreed to get together where she would give me a reading in trade for my helping her. Fortunately, I was quite right, and we cleared up that block in our first session.

Then she delivered the news: When I walked into the bookstore the first day she met me, she told me that Ken had walked in with me (in spirit form). This didn't surprise me actually. What did get my attention, though, was that she now proceeded to pass on very personal information from Ken. For the past year Sharon and I have met weekly, and now my best friend and mentor is with me again as my spirit guide! It doesn't get much better than this. Except it did.

Sharon went on to explain that she has been psychic since childhood, and has a spirit guide named David. Among other things, David was helping her write a book about unconditional love and "the other side of the veil" (the Spirit world). During one of our interactive imagery sessions, Sharon found herself surrounded by a spiritual "presence", was in a complete state of bliss, and was told that she would be "guided to something else." She was to focus on her mediumship and working with "The Veil". It was important that she tell others about this very thin veil that exists between the physical and the spiritual. David and Ken would now be working closely together, and very thankful that they could come through to help us and to give us this information. They had much more to say that needed to go into this book. Once again they were clear, "The truth lies within everyone. Go within and you will know."

At different times when I worked with her, Sharon was able to visit the spiritual plane where Ken is, and was told that we can all go and be there. She had a "HUGE" beautiful image of this realm. Everything is connected in a swirl of energy, and yet there was a stillness where she felt connected to the Core. This Core was a "full spectrum of colors", that had a "musical harmony to it... Everything's being held together as though everything has its own knowing where it's supposed to be. It's staying right there because it knows." She said the experience took her breath away.

Our spirit guides told us many things, including that the soul is only using the physical body for the purpose of experience and learning. We're never alone; angels and spirits are always there to help. True sin is the denial of our Divinity and relationship with the Divine. We were often encouraged to meditate and learn who we really are: "Find the love within."

On September 24, 2008, someone identifying himself as John (different from Shelly's John) began to speak. Sharon set herself aside for him to use her physical voice. Like David and Ken, John began to share his spiritual wisdom. He encouraged my questions. I'd like to share with you some of the questions and answers from our sessions. Then I've asked John to write something to conclude this book.

Chapter 10 - Questions and Answers

September 24, 2008

Dean: Who is speaking (though Sharon)? Are you in a sense like Abraham for Esther and Jerry Hicks?

John: Yes

Dean: So, it's a collective wisdom/consciousness?

John: Yes. We have a vibrational level that will be tuned for her (Sharon), and her only. She's not to channel for just anyone. She will receive information as she progresses. We have a lot to come through. And we'll be more than happy to share with you. There will be a group of us, but John will be the head of our group.

Dean: And John is simply, again, a name or a way to refer to this collective consciousness?

John: John's vibrational level is in a match with Sharon's. And we will speak to John, and he will receive our information and give it to her. She is a good match to John. Just as you have a match, and can receive information, we have chosen Sharon to match up with John.

Dean: So, when Ken and I worked together, and we had what we called mentors and Master Teachers, John is not to be considered as a mentor or Master Teacher in the same way as Ken and I did this? It's more like an "Abraham"?

John: Yes. We are so close, and have so much to give. This is an important time for this information to come through. The world is in oneness with each and every one of us. She is going through pain. Mother Earth has been depleted. Her economics have been depleted. Humanity's spiritual values are the lowest they've ever been. We are here to help turn this around. Mother's soul is withering. Your investments are withering. Your spirituality is withering. You will be brought down to your knees. And then the time will come for rebuilding. We are coming to rebuild her soul, and to put spirituality back before everything withers. It's vital. We've come in multitudes.

Dean: The Mayan calendar suggests that dramatic change is coming in terms of a greater spirituality and less materiality or greed. Is that true?

John: Yes. It's time for humanity to quit taking, and to start giving. High men will be brought down to their knees. Civilization will become more harmonious. There are men in high places that will save this economic condition that you are in, but you are holding on by such a thin thread. Just barely. This is caused from greed.

Dean: Please give us more information.

John: We know you are writing a book. And Ken is very pleased with the work in the book. You have chosen this path before you came down here. There have been so many belief systems out there, and not one is positively correct. But each and every person knows in his heart of Spirit, how important it is to know from whence they've come, and what they are about to be doing, and where they are going. If from your book, you could get just one person who lacks a spiritual connection to really understand the concept of what it means to love oneself, and their value to us on the other side of the veil – these spiritual connections are necessary in order to bring the change that is coming for everyone. Do you not see we are real? That we are so close? Dean, do you not feel our presence?

Dean: Sometimes.

John: Will you put that in your book?

Dean: Yes, I'm going to.

John: Do you bear testimony to the things you have knowledge of in your book?

Dean: Some of it.

John: You have proven yourself, Dean, through Ken, and for Sharon to do this. We will answer your questions. Please be prepared for the next visit.

Dean: Good. Great. If I were to pose one question now: Why does love heal?

Why Love Heals

John: It's because of the vibration of love. It's the energy that is attached to love that heals. Love is the vibration of the soul. It's a direct connection from us on the other side to their soul. It's not a physical connection; it's a spiritual connection. Love is spiritual. Love is a communication, a vibration within itself, a vibration that penetrates to the soul on a soul level. The soul has a different vibration than the physical vibration. Once you've healed and touched the soul, then the body will follow. That's why it's so important for us to have this communication, because through this communication John can touch Sharon's soul, and we can communicate soul to soul. That is how we communicate. That is how Abraham communicates. He is a vibrational level of Esther and Jerry. And this vibration that comes from John and Abraham is an understanding and a knowing of the soul level.

Love touches the soul. The soul is only here in this lifetime temporarily, and then comes back to us. The sweet vibration and harmony of the love that comes through the other side is temporarily forgotten. Once you experience love, true love, there's an automatic, immense realization and knowing of whence you've come. It's a healing. It's a rhythm. It's a knowing. It's an understanding, an awareness. It's a soul level, Dean. There are so many other vibrations that are soul levels that you have not even experienced on this plane.

Joy, you talk about joy, Dean. Joy is a vibration that touches the soul. Just as love is. You were wrong with your book about joy. It was too clinical, Dean. If you had put more experiences of the meaning of joy, then you would have had people reach the vibrational level of joy. Perhaps you could put that joy and love in your next book. There are so many different soul vibrations, Dean, which we will bring to you, so you can put them in as a testament to the vibrations of the great love that is on the other side of the veil that is here for us as well as for you. We progress on the other side of the veil, just as you progress where you are. It is important to us to have these communications. My communication with you, Dean, is at a soul level. It is important that what you need to get across are the vibrations that truly touch the soul. You're here to bring the soul vibrations down to earth. We will bring them down through you, and you will write of them. You have more books to write than what you've written now. The next book you write will be even greater... you will be writing of Truths. Put your soul in your work, Dean.

Dean: Nothing is more important to me than connecting with Spirit and Truth... I don't make excuses for being clinical to start with in my book. That was my background, and what I thought I needed to do. I'm willing to relay your message, and talk from my personal experience... I think this is going to be fun.

John: Don't think we weren't with you when you wrote your first book. The things in your first book were to be said, and the way that you put it. We love you dearly, Dean. Your second book will be different. And your third book will be different from the first two. You'll be seeing the progress as you go. You will see the changes that you will be making – just different information coming in a different form. You have opened up this channel, and we are so pleased. Do you not see that your first book was what it was to be at the time? And now your second book will be even more spiritual... Your audience has been prepared for you and your book. It's the times, Dean. People's spirits are being moved now. Their hearts are being receptive to the things that you have to give them. We have prepared you, and we have prepared them. We will point the way for you. We will open doors for you. Be patient. Finish the second book. Your trust and loyalty have been proven. Again, before I go, you must know of our love for you and Shelly, and for those you come in contact with. You are where you're supposed to be, and doing what you're supposed to be doing. Please leave the door to your home open. We shall continue to open your hearts to those who we will bring to both of you.

Dean: It's a deal.

John: Thank you, Dean. Thank you, Shelly. Thank you.

October 9, 2008

Dean: One of the things I've come to believe that is at the core of why we're here, is to love ourselves, to love all, everything. And if we really knew who we were in terms of Divinity/One with God – then everything goes pretty well. But it seems that the "field experience" of human life in a sense forces us to look within, to find love within, because we're not finding it outside as such. Is there truth in that?

John: Yes, in fact, Dean, the truth is that you knew that you were to come down here. This is not about worthiness or trying to pass a test. Indeed, this is to find joy. This is to experience joy. It's something that you have to experience on a vibrational level for you to gain the knowledge that is needed to be able to hold the vibration of love. Without experiencing some form or the different forms of love, then you do not understand or will not be able to reconnect with that vibration from The Source. You have chosen to come down here to gain joy, to gain freedom, but also a remembrance of the vibrations that were on the other side of the veil.

There was a veil drawn between you and this experience of this plane. The reasons for the veil are several, but it is to create a loss of memory for the vibrations that you are to connect to on this side. Just as there are many values to the light spectrum, there are many values to energy. When you're born here, you were born with unknowing of this spectrum, this source. However, when you're born you have that within yourself. Using the experiences here on this plane, you will begin to understand and feel and gain knowledge of who you truly are. We want you to enjoy this life plane. And through the joy of these different vibrations and experiences, you will learn what love truly is. Love is not the most important thing on this plane, but will simply allow you to experience a relationship with those vibrations of the different sources of love. Those sources of love you can only experience on this physical plane. As you evolve, and as we have evolved, we have not only enjoyed the experiences of vibrations of love on your planet, but we have moved on and progressed and have gained knowledge of other vibrations of love at a different intensity.

You have old beliefs that must be made new. And this is the purpose of your book, Dean – to let people know that once they experience joy through music, through song, through listening to the waterfall, through meditation, that this joy would move them to the next vibration, which is then the vibration of love. You can't just be love. You must program or experience the joy, and then experience the love, experience the knowledge, experience the intensity, and so forth. Growth – you came down here to grow, Dean. You cannot grow without experience. You agreed to come down and experience the different vibrations on this plane. One of those vibrations is joy. When you move through the vibration of joy, you will see that it has different fingers coming out of it, or different paths – a path of joy going up towards the vibration of love, or a path going through the pure simplicity of just enjoying nature.

There are other types of joy – of seeing a first-born baby, and so on and so forth. Through the different experiences you then learn the different experiences of love – the love of your mother, your wife, the love of your dog, the love of the sunshine, and so forth. Even the love of nature is a different vibration. All these different vibrations from love, which you will need to experience through the journey on this plane, will help you to evolve, and help those sisters and brothers around you who are like-minded, and even those who are not like-minded, to be able to move on their pathway of evolution. This is a continuous evolution in eternity. But what is most important right now, Dean, is first to accept the experience of joy. Children feel the joy; the first emotion is joy for them, not the love of their father or mother.

It's through their care and understanding and their experiences that they either come to love or to become displeased with what is going on in their life. Joy is a natural, normal vibration that we're all in tune with, and connect to on the other side of the veil. That joy has been brought through to you, and is your first experience.

Dean: Well, that being said, then *Doctor's Orders: Go Fishing* was hardly an accidental message: Follow your bliss.

John: As Sharon would say, you've hit the nail on the head.

Dean: You said that our first experience here is joy, which can lead to love (or not). So, the additional benefit of experience and growth is that we need "contrast" as a way to help us more fully appreciate what love is. We need to experience what love is not in order to more fully appreciate what love is. So, it's all beneficial, and ideally we learn the easier way through joy and wonder and awe rather than looking for love in all the wrong places and then having to be driven or forced inside, to look within to find that love?

John: That is correct. Thank you, Dean.

Dean: I appreciate this. You know me – the perfectionist part – I've got to be right. But I want to tell the truth. And I feel so very, very fortunate that you're willing to use me, and let me do this. I enjoy this.

John: Dean, you asked for this position before you came down here. Your meeting with Sharon was no accident. Your meeting with Ken was no accident. You have been prepared, and you agreed, before you came down, to experience both the negative and positive, so that you can experience true joy. That connection with your decision to come down here will reign through you. Your experiences of joy and your vibrational level that has come down here has brought people to your life for this very purpose of writing these books.

Dean: In reading the Esther Hicks' books, a strong statement is made, also, that we need to experience contrast as a way to constantly make decisions or preferences, which adds to the constant growth and expansion of the universe – that it's simply essential for the growth and expansion of the universe.

John: That is correct. But, let me again tell you that the contrast comes through your choice. The freedom is given to you while you're here on this plane to choose what experiences that you will have. There was not a plan laid out for you that says that you will choose to be this or that, or you're going to choose to be loving or to feel anger. Those were your choices, your free agency to gain the knowledge that you need to continue to evolve.

Dean: However, when you say that we are not coming in to experience certain things as such, it seems like the plan is laid out enough that it isn't accidental or so hit and miss.

John: It's important for you to understand that you set the plan prior to coming down here – the things that you wanted to experience. Yes, this is true, but we want you to understand the importance of free agency. Whether your plan was preordained, we have given you the gift of making those choices down here. Intuition, feelings, and synchronicities will acknowledge that you are on the path that you previously chose to come through. But if you do not choose that path while you're here, you can come back and experience it again at a later time. It is so important that you understand that while you're here you can choose a different path. If you're in alignment with the vibrations prior to coming here, you will notice that you will be in tune with your intuition and your synchronicities and your dreams. But it is not about proving yourself or an idea of having to gain certain experiences. It is so vital to understand that these experiences will come to you sooner or later.

Dean: So, Ken taught me that we come into a particular life experience, and bring in certain things we've learned and things we want to learn more. The way I say it is, the script is written, but how well you play the part is the difference. So, the scriptwriters, including you and me and whomever, have come together in preplanning a particular life experience. We say here is the role, and you've demonstrated certain things that would benefit this role. But there are some other things that you need to learn, that would expand you or help you grow as the actor. And, so, you simply in the most loving way come in and have this wonderful opportunity to act with the greatest joy and enthusiasm and interest, and hopefully play it to your satisfaction.

John: Yes.

Dean: Cool.

Dean: If there is a life plan or pre-planning, if there is a law of attraction and this is a participatory universe, and if we are directly responsible for all of our thoughts and feelings, when and why is there ever Divine intervention?

John: Hmmm, Dean, do you not understand that you came down here with Divine intervention? That is another side of humanity. You have never lacked touch with Divine intervention. There was no beginning when you came down here, or a separation of the Divine intention. You are Divine. You are co-creating what you truly desire from a soul's standpoint. Your spiritual guides, like Ken, vibrate at the same level that you do. That connection never dissolves. You have within you a vibration that you would say is like DNA, your own private vibration with different harmonies that attuned you to the experiences and the agreements made prior to coming here.

Prior to coming here, you and Ken and your guides and guardian angels all vibrated at the same frequency that is yours or theirs that you agreed to vibrate with. It's about energy and the different levels of energy. Your physical plane has only the ability to vibrate within the levels of this plane. However, your soul vibrations are vibrations of the eternities. At a soul level you are connecting to the vibrations of the universal consciousness. Do you see that the soul vibrations are the vibrations of the universal consciousness, whereas the vibrations that you experience in the physical realm or plane are the vibrations that we are allowing you to experience on this plane? So, as you progress through eternity, you will come back into the realization of the vibrations prior to this plane. You will again attune to, or we might say, have the feeling of coming home. It is a feeling of resonating with the universal vibrations. You will step in and out of these vibrations to experience vibrations on other planes. And as you experience these other vibrations, you will bring that experience back up and into the home of the universal consciousness. The secret is that through the knowledge of joy, is the attachment to love. We tend to think love is, like you said earlier, outside of ourselves. But it isn't. It is who we are. It is our vibration. It is who and what the soul is. The soul is joy seeking knowledge and seeking experience. There are so many more secrets. If people could only vibrate to the level of joy, they could experience the many, many, many facets of love, as the many facets as of a diamond.

Dean: When I talk about the zero point field, or in quantum physics this underlying energy matrix of harmony and order, is that God? Or does the zero point field have all the fundamental aspects of God or spiritual consciousness, but God is always bigger?

John: The zero point field carries with it the aspect of God, the God Source. God is eternally evolving. This zero point is the zero point of Divine Source.

Dean: You're saying this isn't God in that God is always evolving, but it's as close as we're gong to get to understanding God?

John: On this plane. Absolutely.

Dean: Could we essentially define this vibration, or glue of harmony and order that connects everything, as love?

John: The vibration that runs through the universe is an eternal vibration of the cosmos. Only on this physical plane do you have the vibration of contrast to love. So, it would be hard for me to explain to you in the preexistence, or the eternal vibrations, the Divine Source. It is only through your contrast down here on this earthly plane that you experience love and its opposite. You must understand that the source of love comes from the vibration of the source of joy. Love is many vibrations, so it is hard for me to try to understand what vibration you are trying to connect to.

Dean: I'll try again. My understanding is, in terms of quantum physics, that there indeed is oneness – in that if we take the smallest particle and split it, whatever we do to one part instantaneously happens to the other – suggesting a oneness or a connectedness.

John: Absolutely. That connectedness is the vibration of the Divine Source, and flows through every soul on both sides of the veil.

Dean: So, whenever we're resonating with our true essence, we allow the flow of this life force energy, and experience greater ease or health. When we are experiencing separation in any way, we restrict the flow of that life force energy, and then experience the consequences of that.

John: Absolutely. Thank you, Dean.

There is so much information that has been given through Sharon in these conversations with John that we could easily fill another book. I want to add one more piece of information, and then I've asked John to add whatever else he would like to say to conclude this book.

I had asked John to differentiate between one's own intuition, spirit guides, soul, and Divine Source. He explained that our own intuition is connecting with our own soul energy. It has its own memories and experiences and knowledge gained from previous lifetimes, which are guided by the soul's decisions and plans. Divine Source is a different energy level. We need to resonate with pure joy to make this connection to Divine Source. Spirit guides come from our own unique soul group, and have had prior physical life experience/existence. Master teachers have been on higher planes, and have access to more information of different levels and realms. Shelly then asked John, "At what level are you?" John went on to describe his Ascended Master level, and identified himself, "My name is John the Baptist." He went on to say a whole lot more, and completely "blew us away." He has agreed to tell his life story in a next book. His story will be very different than what you've been told.

John the Baptist Speaks

This is where I've asked John to say whatever he would like to say to conclude this book. The remaining pages in this chapter are all his words.

We are so thankful that you have invited us to be a part of this book. It is with great pleasure that we take advantage of this opportunity. Dean has given of himself in working with Sharon, his reputation, and the divine resonating with his "soul print" at this time to bring forth the information in this book. We, again, acknowledge his spirit and his love in his heart for giving of himself and his time. Dean has come through at this time giving great sacrifice. It is important that he has sacrificed his time on this plane, with his sweet wife, adjusting his timetables and his resources to putting this book together for us as well as for you, the reader of this information.

Dear reader, much love comes from the Source of your soul groups that this information is coming through at this time. We are so glad (the universe, all planes, and Mother Earth) that you who are walking on this planetary plane have opened yourself to the raising of the consciousness at this time. You have all committed on the other side of the veil, through your preexistence, to come down here at this time. Enormous multitudes of soul groups have come to join forces with your energy in raising this consciousness with us. There are many of us here at this time: Abraham, the twelve disciples, as well as others, and myself who have come before. We have come back down with you as agreed, to resonate with you, and to join forces with your soul plan and your soul print. And it is through your soul print that we harmonize and resonate with you during this time. We're so eternally grateful for this worldwide collection of energies that has connected with the Source of nature.

Truly the forces of nature and this theme now of the "green" planet (working with recycling, and environmental policies) are all part of the ordained energy that is circling around Mother Earth and vibrating with her. Mother Earth's heat and vibration are transcending throughout nature. Her energy eruptions and magna are putting out much energy, which is coming through the trees, the atmosphere, the weather, the water; there is much connection with the oneness of us all.

It is so important that this universal connection and this oneness be put out through your prayers and through your connection with nature. Feel this energy spinning around Mother Earth, and a connection with her gravitational forces that are holding you closer to her at this time. Just as there is no hatred in animals, or no sin in the animals on this earth, there is no animosity in our weather, or in any form of nature. It is important that humanity begins to raise its energy to the pure energies of nature, and can feel that Divine energy. Can you evolve closer to nature, and bring nature into your homes and your apartments? Can you push back the cement, the blacktopping, and the confinement of what you're doing to our Mother Earth? You are confining her. She needs her free agency, her freedom to expand. You are taking this expansion away from her, and, also, your own free agency away from yourselves. And by taking this freedom, you are also disconnecting yourself from the true love that is there. Oh, we are so grateful for Dean and this book to be put out so you can connect to your Divine Love Source.

Please reach out and use the energy, your own creativity, the political energy, the energy of the universe, to step up at this time, and to make commitments to connect with this Divine Source. There will be much coming through your connecting. Energies are going to be sped up. You will be vibrating at a higher level because without your help not only will there be great commotion on your planet, but can you see and feel the pain that will be sent throughout your solar system? The need to connect with Divine Source at this time is great. It is extremely important that the consciousness of this universe be raised. It can only be raised one at a time through your own resonating with this Divine Source Energy.

This is the time that you need to see who you are. You truly are the Divine Source of Love. We have asked to work with Dean for this book. Can you not see the importance of this book? It is bringing through this great connection with Divine Source Love. This connection will be out there for those who want to make this commitment, connection, and the ability to use this energy for the eternal evolvement of this universe. Things will begin to speed up for all of you, and much creation and evolvement is going to come through your internet, your connection with other planets and other worlds, and other beings. Time is being sped up, and it is so important, and we are so grateful for these connections. We are also looking forward to the next writing, Dean's next book, and more information that will be coming through.

It's important to understand that you truly are Divine Source. And as being Divine Source, you have the attachment to the energy of love. You need to become aware of this energy source – that it resides within everyone. While you're here on this physical plane, you are experiencing many emotions. Love is one of those emotions. However, emotions like sorrow, pain and fear, only reside here on this physical plane. Love is the one energy that goes from the solar plexus to the heart, and

then to the true Divine Source of which you are. The other emotions are not attached, or are not a part of the energy that is attached to Divine Source. So, you see that while we're in the physical body, we, not realizing who we are (that we are Divine), come on this plane focused on the physical body and the physical plane. We attach to and identify ourselves with our physical self, and to the physical emotions.

So, as we grow, we become at war with these emotions. We do not love them for what they are. Once people realize that they are more than their physical body, and can get to the point where they realize that they are all one Spirit of Divine Source or Divine Energy, then they truly can touch and be a part of that Source of God. And while we are busy warring within ourselves, sometimes we reach out and war with others, and the strife and the turmoil gets going, and we have war within our communities, then within the governments and nations, and pretty soon that energy is felt worldwide. Not everyone wants to take the responsibility of owning that energy, and the relationship that they must have with this energy. It is also of great importance for people to realize that the source of the energy comes from within. They have separated themselves from the energy of Divine Source. So, it is important that they come in contact with any type of spiritual source.

All on the earth plane have their own source and way of connecting to Spirit. The importance is to make the contact with Divine Source. When people misperceive the truth of who they are, they separate their physical self from Divine Source, and they look for a guru, somebody outside of themselves, instead of looking within. If they could truly see themselves, and trust themselves, and honor each and every one of their emotions, and learn to love each emotion.

Research the emotion of hate and what it is that you hate, and understand where the hate is coming from. It is okay to hate, to have sorrow, and to feel pain. You must go in and become friends with the pain. You need to acknowledge the pain or the hate or the sorrow or the torment. What part of the physical body is this energy coming from? You need to realize that these emotions are an important part of your being, and understand what this emotion has to say for you, for your healing process, and to be able to reconnect with this emotion through love. Then you are connecting that solar plexus energy to the heart energy, and the heart energy is the true connection to Divine Source.

This is a difficult process, but is a process that we accepted in the preexistence. We, being full of Divine Source and God-like energy, thought that our Divine Source energy was strong enough, and truly is strong enough, to overcome the physical emotions and struggles, and pains of the body as well. It's just that we give in and allow the physical energy to separate and to overpower the God Source. We do not realize that the miracle of life is truly coming from the God Source. Through experiences such as lovemaking and great ecstasy with our partner, and experiences of pure creativity that are deeply felt within, we touch the energy of our heart. This source of joy and passion and harmony is one of the closest times we're connected truly with the Divine Source. This is when we're acting as co-creators bringing more of that Divine Energy Source onto this plane.

We chose in the preexistence to perceive a separation through our daily lives, through illnesses, or whatever trigger factors there are out there, in order to grow. Your growth and what you truly came down to experience is not to learn to hate, to have sorrow, to learn to have pain or to learn to be tormented on this plane. What you truly came down for was to feel in a physical body the different types of energies so that you could make peace with them, and to realize there is always that Eternal Connection.

On this plane there is much talk about oneness. Oneness is extremely important because oneness comes from the energy of Divine Source. Once we bring those who are on this physical plane back in alignment to the oneness of the source of Godness, of True Love, True Source, then come the miracles – the miracles of healing, the miracles of transformation, the miracles of connectedness to all that is here on this plane. The most natural source of oneness and Divine Source on this physical plane is through nature. So, you see how easy it would be through nature to connect to that Divine Source. We did not bring you down here, nor did you come, thinking that you would be separate from Spirit. We are all here walking with you, and guiding you in your dreams, through synchronicities, through your guides and your angels, and the angels of nature, the angel of the dogs, the rabbits, the nature of the waterfall, and the nature of flowers. That beauty is here telling you as loudly as we can that you are surrounded in everything you do and see with loving energy – with the sunlight, the moonlight, and the universal energies. If people could only take the focus off of themselves, their separateness and self-centeredness, and could go in and see that eternal connection that they have within themselves. They would then see that they truly are physical, as well as spiritual beings, and see their spiritual connection and evolution.

There have been many masters sent to earth: Muhammad, Jesus, Buddha. Many master teachers have been here, and there will continue to be teachers coming, like Abraham, myself, and others who will be here working. The time is coming quickly; the universal consciousness is coming closer and closer. There is urgency about making the shift that is coming. The shifts have come in their own time, and are a part of the universal network or timing. As we get closer and closer to this source of energy that is coming to heal all, including our Mother Earth, the importance of making peace is a part of the survival of this solar system.

We are all connected to a universal source of energy. Even the stars bring a higher vibrational energy that is truly connected to the God Source energy. Can everyone not see that this Loving Source surrounds this earth? Can you not see that you have separated yourselves from this loving Source? The veil is so very, very thin. Sharon knows of the thinness of the veil, and so desires to be able to walk back and forth through it because she is so connected to this spiritual plane. So is everyone else. But she is also so connected to David, who radiates this Divine Source energy. She does not know the true source of the energy. However, when she goes in and creates the relationship between her and David, she connects to this Divine Source.

Many people connect to this Divine Source through prayers. That is the closest they come to the reality within themselves that they truly can connect by themselves through opening up, and allowing themselves to see themselves as the Divine Rose that is but a bud. And as *they become awakened to the beauty and the Divine Spirit within – as their petals open up, and they begin to pass the constriction of warring within themselves – they become more in love with themselves. It is all a part of what they are to experience.*

It's natural and normal, and part of the physical humanness to feel all that they feel, but not to continue to war within themselves. As they honor all of their feelings they slowly begin to love themselves, and to see that the past was part of what they were to go through. They must understand that they can only love that past through the love that they give it in the present. You can only give love in the present. You cannot give love to a past circumstance by going back and saying I love that experience. You must go back to the experience and feel the torment, and then love that torment because, oh yes, that was you in your humanness. Accept what is. Love what is. Trust what is.

Do you understand the process of the opening of the flower? That within each and every one of us there are petals that need to be opened? And as people open the petals themselves, they can only do that in their present state. The emotion that is attached to the past must be opened and experienced and given the loving energy that it needs to experience. And the energy must be truly felt and nurtured with an acceptance that this is a normality that each and every one of us will feel at one time or another in our life.

That is another part of our interconnectedness. We are all going to experience these different emotions at different times, and through different avenues in our life. We need to accept that this is a normal reality, and that we must look at that, bring awareness to that, and love the fact that we have experienced that emotion, and the importance to experience it in both a negative as well as a positive way. Once we take that negative vibration and understand its purpose on this the planetary plane, then we will know that we are to give it love, and thank it for coming in and giving us the opportunity for that experience. If we do not acknowledge and give gratitude for that opportunity to experience these emotions through the different modalities that they come through, our progression or growth will be hampered.

So, with giving thanks to that petal one at a time, as it unfolds, and releasing the constriction of the bud, the gentle sunlight comes through, the light of Divine Source comes through, and warms that beautiful rose. With its Divine connection to that energy, it will open truly loving all of those experiences. Each petal will unfold at its own time, and in the harmonies or in the sequence that the petals on a rose normally unfold. They do not unfold all at once, but one at a time in their gentleness, and with love, always facing toward the source of light, knowing that it is Divine, and where its source and energy comes from.

This rose is very much planted on this universe in its dirt with all the trials and troubles that it takes within itself to find its nutrients, its water, and its sustenance in order to bring forth the beauty of itself, its oneness. It takes a great deal for that to happen. And as it is growing and becoming, it also has thorns.

Now, this rose has earned those thorns, and shows all that the thorns are something that is part of its evolution, and must be a part of it while it is growing toward Divine Energy. But this rose knows that from the time it was planted, that it truly was, and contained, Divine Source. Once that rose opens, and gives out its true beauty, and its physical being, its aroma, its gratefulness, its love for itself, and for the thorns, and for what it has gone through – the rose still is and always will be beautiful.

This is what humans are. Humans are always, and will always be connected to Divine Source, the source of love of God. Humans will always be love. Humans must experience emotions (both positive and negative) on this side of the veil in order to grow. They must learn to love the growth that they have gone through. It is important to go back with awareness and understand where the emotion came from, and then love the experience or synchronicity or coincidence that surrounded that emotion. Accept it as normal and what one is to experience. Love both the negative growth of it, as well as the positive.

If they could just only do this one simple task – to truly learn to love and forgive the negative. And if they could truly love that, and go through a daily ritual, or a daily awareness, or a daily task that brings them back into remembrance of who they are, Dean, this is the greatest message I would want to give.

Chapter 11 - Final Thoughts

I realize I said that John the Baptist's words would conclude this book. I almost feel like I'm committing some kind of sin to have asked John for his contribution, and then add my own human thoughts and words. What could I possibly say or add? Actually, what follows is something I wanted to include in the book all along. This allows me to reemphasize a point of great importance.

John just said that remembering who we truly are was his greatest message. We are one with All That Is. And as we live our lives in harmony with our Source, we will know a greater ease, peace of mind, and grow spiritually. This is the message of all the great Masters, religions, and spiritual systems. Now I ask your indulgence to let me tell one more story. In truth, it's Gloria Wendroff's story.

Gloria describes herself as someone who throughout her life was not particularly spiritual or religious. But she had a few unique transcendent experiences that gradually transformed her life. She had always wanted to be a writer, and was a literature major in college. Once, while writing a story, she said "it was like another voice took over... it was like the story was writing itself." This would lead to what she calls "Godwriting" and "Heaven Letters".

Later in her life, while meditating, she had a personal revelation that she was a spiritual being. She said she found that her desire to know God heightened, and "In loneliness and wanting and wondering and doubting and ignorance, I asked my human questions, and answers came." After yet another "spiritual awakening" experience, Christ appeared to her and said that he had been seeking her, which left her dumbfounded. Then she had the clear insight that "the seeker and the sought are the same." We are all one with God.

She considered herself a most unlikely person to have had this experience. Yet now she was being asked to spread God's word through her teaching and writing. Daily, what she calls God – a "Voiceless Voice that captures my being" - talks with, and through her. It's like God is whispering thoughts, and she's listening for them. "Godwriting is the process of listening to the Voice within, and having your own one-on-one communication with God." Everyone can hear God's words; "all it takes is desire, the asking, and the listening."

Every day Gloria emails her "dictated" inspirational messages from God, what she calls, "Heaven Letters". I have received and read these letters daily for the past year. I heard about them through Dr. Bernie Siegel, who says that he reads them each morning, and forwards them to physicians and friends regularly. I find them truly inspirational. You can find them, and her story, on her website (www.heavenletters.org). You can also find them compiled in her book, *Heaven Letters, Love Letters from God, Book One*, (the forward is by Bernie Siegel). Here's one of my favorites, titled, "Multiply God's Joy".

God said:
Come to Me like butterflies. Let Me be the nectar you drink. Come to Me like butterflies. Fly around Me. Alight on Me. Come as one, or come as many. The thing is to come to Me. Flock around Me. Surround

Me with your love. Can you imagine My joy in butterflies? Multiply My joy.

Can you imagine My joy in you? Would you deny Me even one moment of joy? Would you deny Me anything I ask? Would you deny Me you?

I am under your spell, and I hold you in My thrall.

Who leads and who follows? Who is in front when no one is behind? All I want is to be with you, and with you I AM. I am your Host and I am your Guest. I serve and am served. I am your Waiter and you are Mine.

There is nothing to say. There is everything to be. There isn't anything that We are not. We are the table and We are the chairs. We are the people who sit in the chairs, and We are the food on the table. We are the food about to be eaten, and We are the food eaten.

We turn somersaults in the air, and We land in Heaven.

We turn the world upside down. We write in the sand. We write on water, We wear down the rocks with our love. We build mountains, and We take them apart.

We polish the stars and look at Ourselves in them.

We hug the moon, and We enter the sun. We do a jig and find Ourselves in a tree that We are the fruit of, and We nibble on Ourselves.

We return to the good earth, and We dig deep. Everywhere We find treasure, untold treasure. We take it out, and We leave it there. Let someone else find it. There is more where that came from.

The biggest treasure is the treasure within. That's where We matter most. This is where We find Ourselves. We are valiant and untrodden there. We hold each other tight as We do not hold at all. The magnet of love keeps us together. All the colors of love douse us, and We are sparkled. From the depths of soul We rise. We rise and We stay. We go everywhere, and never leave. We multi-task the Universe. We are everywhere all at once, and yet there is nowhere to be. Space is not. Time is not.

There is no place to be, and no when to be there. All greet Us, and yet no one is there, and no one arrives. All are seated somewhere or in bed.

Are We in a mirage or a miracle? And Who cares? What is the difference when We are love, and We stand on Our tiptoes reaching high and bending low to pick everyone up?

What is the difference between sense and nonsense when We are just passing time, as it were, even as We are not in time and never out of it?

How can We get closer, when there is no closer to get? And yet I say, "Come

closer. Come closer to Me. Fly to Me like
Butterflies. Waft around Me."

Whom am I talking to? What do
butterflies want with words when love will
do, when love will do better?

Who cares about words when that
which words represent is better, far better,
and yet presently, We would be at a loss
without words. And yet We have them, and
We use them, and yet love needs no words
and has nothing to do with vocabulary.

I recommend that you attend her "Godwriting"
workshop. Here she demonstrates that we all have clear
and easy access to Divine guidance and wisdom. This is
what I have been taught through Ken's and my spiritual
guides and teachers all along. Gloria's story reminds me,
and compels me, to tell you how accessible God or Divine
Source is. I have been told consistently, "I am closer than
a breath away".

Gloria's story also brings to mind the story of Neale
Donald Walsch, and his conversations with God, which I
mentioned in Chapter 9. I've always loved his story and
the messages in his books. Like Gloria, he understood that
the information he was given was meant for everyone,
which was why he wrote the books.

Do you remember the 1977 movie, *Oh, God!*,
staring John Denver, Terri Garr, and George Burns? John
was the unlikely supermarket manager chosen by God to
spread his message. He was so reluctant. How could this
be true? Why would God choose him? The message, of
course, is that God is here always for everyone. "Red and

yellow, black and white, we are precious in his sight". Everyone, without exception!

I have to admit that I've felt a bit like Gloria, Neale, and John Denver at times. Connecting with Spirit is a truly unique experience. It has been a revelation that I greatly relish and treasure. But it's one thing to have this very personal experience, and it's quite another to share it publicly. I've already mentioned this earlier regarding transcendent experiences. You don't want your story diminished.

I talk with Spirit through my intuition. I have been surely blessed also that I can talk with spirit guides and teachers through Ken's and Sharon's ability to channel this wisdom. There is nothing that I value more. Yet I realize that not everyone will understand or accept my experience or beliefs. And this is as it should be. We need to respect our individual differences. When will we know everything there is to know about a particular subject, or any subject? Indeed, this raises the question: How do we determine the truth of anything?

I encourage you to trust your own experience. Of course, we can also look to science. But my experience has taught me also to look inside. Every philosophical and spiritual system throughout history has told us that the truth lies within us. People have always known and been taught that they have a deep sense of belonging to Spirit. It is who we are.

It is easy to become focused on the physical. We are most certainly a physical body and perceive life through our physical senses. But, in fact, as the saying goes, we are spiritual beings having a physical experience. More accurately, we are spiritual beings having a spiritual experience. Who we are is not confined to our human bodies because the soul has no boundaries. Our soul uses the physical body for the purpose of experience and learning. As the apostle Paul stated, "We are in the world, but not of it."

Joan Borysenko addresses this issue eloquently in her book, *Guilt is the Teacher, Love is the Lesson.* She writes that enlightenment is the self-realization of our "faulty identification with our ego roles." Who we are is "a more basic, enduring identity:"

> In Self-realization, our personality –
> our ego – is seen as no more and no less
> important than the identity we have chosen
> to accomplish our unique work in the
> world. It's great to have a personality, all
> right, but it is no more "us" than the clothes
> we hang over the back of our chair when we
> go to bed at night.

I also strongly agree with Joan Borysenko in her book, *Your Soul's Compass.* She and her coauthor, Gordon Dveirin, consulted 27 Sages from diverse wisdom traditions, asking what is the nature of spiritual guidance. Why are we here? What is life's purpose? They found that there was one universal experience regardless of the religious or spiritual belief system: the Mystic Heart. It coincided with the message of Brother Wayne Teasdale, to whom they dedicated their book. The Truth of who we are and why we're here is found through the practice of meditation or related transcendent experience. This is when the Mystic Heart emerges, and we connect with our Divine Source.

In his book, *The Mystic Heart: Discovering Universal Spirituality in the World's Religions*, Teasdale claims that all religion arises out of mystical experience. He encourages people to discover (or rediscover) the contemplative roots and practices of their specific religion. He promotes a universal spirituality based on compassion, which he calls "interspirituality".

There's a fascinating video dialogue between Teasdale and Ken Wilbur that I recommend you see, which you can find on the Internet (www.in.integralinstitute.org). Here, Teasdale discusses his concept of the mystic heart and its practical implications. I love the way he attempts to explain God and who we are:

> Imagine, if you will, a large board that has holes in it, thousands of holes, through which light can come – and that is this side of existence that we're in now. On the other side of the board, is an infinitely infinite light. And this infinitely infinite light is pure consciousness itself – undifferentiated, unconditioned, totally aware, Sat Chit Ananda, Nirvana, the infinite reality... with an infinite number of attributes, with that deep intention of love. That's God and Godhead... the active and the passive... And we are those little points of light.

If we could only open up to this truth of who we are. We are love itself. We are God manifesting in physical form. God, love, and Divine Consciousness is all there is. There is no separation from Divine Source. We are God-stuff, perfect in every way.

<u>My Truth</u>

Picture two lines together perfectly parallel. Then imagine them moving and waving together in perfect synchrony. Whatever one line does, the other does at the precise moment of the other. In fact, there is no way to determine which line moves first. They both follow each other, or follow some invisible force that conducts them in total harmony.

Now imagine a bunch of lines moving, waving and vibrating in similar form. All peak and trough, move up and down, in absolute unison. These wavelengths can be all sizes, large and small, but all are perfectly aligned. All are singing and dancing and moving as one.

This is a way to begin to understand the unity that underlies all of creation. At the most fundamental level, all atomic and subatomic matter work and exist in harmony and order. Everything is interconnected and functions as one.

This is how our bodies work, as well, when they're healthy. Most of the time the trillions and trillions of cells in our bodies work together in unbelievable harmony. They cooperate beautifully to keep us breathing, living, growing, and thriving.

When we do things like eating nutrient-rich foods and exercising our muscles in appropriate balance, it contributes to the harmony and growth of our cells. When we are joyful and "going fishing", this emotional state also resonates with the natural harmony of our cells and contributes to our health. When we are practicing wellness, all the electrons that comprise our bodies are dancing together in the greatest line dance you could ever imagine. Think trillions and trillions of Fred Astaires and Ginger Rogers waltzing and spinning and swaying as one.

However, when we experience chaos or dissonance or stress, the harmonious movement and activity of the cells is disrupted. When we eat something that is not able to be properly absorbed and used by our cells – and when we don't exercise our muscles appropriately – and when we experience "negative" emotions – all of these cause the vibration of our cells to not be able to dance the same dance in harmony. The cells can then weaken, and the systems in our bodies stop operating optimally. Disease is now able to thrive in the environment of our bodies, where normally it would be sitting out the dance.

So, back to my recent comments that we are God and love itself. We are an aspect of God manifesting in physical form, and connected through Divine Consciousness to every other aspect of All That Is. Let me also remind you of the core virtues of wisdom and knowledge, courage, humanity (which includes love), justice, temperance, and transcendence (which includes beauty, gratitude, hope, humor, and spirituality). The reason why these virtues are so valued is because they are in resonance with who we are at the deepest level.

When we express or experience these virtues, it's like getting a "tune up." For example: Remember in science class when iron filings were scattered on a card held over a magnet? They always arranged themselves in the pattern of the "lines of force" of the magnet's field. Similarly, love functions like a magnet's force field, and realigns the molecules of our bodies with their fundamental, natural state of harmony and order. The feelings and vibrations generated by love and all virtues are a resonant energy that is absorbed, aligns, and delivers everything the body or soul needs to function with peak performance. It's the perfect remedy or prescription. This is why love heals.

The quantum field, Life Force, and Qi energy described in ancient wisdom texts, are all ways to label or understand the fundamental "glue" of the universe that flows through and connects everything. When you are aligned or resonating with this energy matrix of harmony and order, you allow for a greater flow of this life-giving energy through your body.

Love is the natural, inherent energy of the universe. It is in fact, our True Self. We are the Holy Grail we've been looking for. We are so inclined to look for love, and anything we think will make us feel better, but we're looking in all the wrong places. We can find quick, short-term fixes through any number of addictions, but anything that is not on the same wavelength as unconditional love and compassion is just not going to cut it long-term.

Band-aids don't and won't cure chronic disease. You must deal with what has created the dissonance that underlies the symptoms of heart disease, cancer, strokes, diabetes, etc. Medications or pharmaceuticals are attempts to restore a chemical balance in the body. But if we don't address what is restricting the flow of the quantum or Life Force energy, our symptoms will persist. Our symptoms truly are the signal or benevolent messenger that something is resisting our connection with Divine Source or God.

This is why I love the message of *Doctor's Orders: Go Fishing* – the need to bring more joy into our lives. This is why the will to live is curative. Joy is a resonant energy of our soul or True Self. And when you heal the soul, the body follows.

The key is to get the cells of the body back to vibrating as one. Love is the expression or experience of oneness – this is why love is defined as oneness. Love expressed as listening, caring, compassion, hope, etc. literally bathes the cells of your body with exactly what they need to return to their natural state of oneness.

Meditation and various forms of prayer or focused attention are also ways to enable the flow of the Life Force. Meditating and connecting with your soul's energy and Divine Consciousness are always sound prescriptions for health and healing. This is why meditation has been a primary practice throughout the ages. And this is why love has been taught as the ultimate life practice and attainment. Love is the most life-enhancing experience we can have. It is always healing and restorative.

I'm very pleased through this book to present you my truth and my story. I pray it reminds and encourages you to resonate with your own truth – the truth of who you really are.

Remember my diagnostic code of "Forgotten Identity". This is our greatest ailment. The cure is to reconnect with our Divinity. When we resonate with our core essence of love – well-being is the only outcome. This is why love heals.

Believe me, I know that this isn't that easy. It's simple, but it isn't easy. Our soul's journey is to experience "contrast" in order to understand love more fully. As crazy as it may seem, we have purposely chosen to experience what love is not, so that we can appreciate more fully what love is – in a way we're not soon to forget.

Think about it. If you were to reflect back on your life, and what you value the most, it's likely to include the "hard times." The times you grew in understanding, knowledge, wisdom, and satisfaction were learned in "the school of hard knocks". You wouldn't necessarily choose to go back and re-experience these tough times, but you wouldn't choose to give up what you've learned as a result. As we get older we can wish to have our youth again. But I doubt that you would trade your learned wisdom for youth. You'd only go back to being young again if you could take what you've learned with you. These are the things you will savor and remember through the eternities. This all contributes to your spiritual growth.

So, let me remind you to be easier on yourself. You are not judged. Life is not a test. You are not born in sin. You are never alone. But you will need faith and courage as you face the daily trials and limitations of life in the physical. This is why John the Baptist ended the last chapter asking us to love and forgive the negative. And to go through some daily ritual that will remind us of who we are and why we're here. When you're in the middle of a tornado, you're not likely thinking that this is an opportunity for spiritual growth. It's easy to get distracted and forget our connection to Spirit.

One of the things I do that helps me remember, and stay connected, is the Heaven Letters I receive in an email everyday. My wife also has Doreen Virtue's "Healing With the Angels" cards. Each morning we pick and read a card for an inspirational message to carry with us through the day. Of course, I also meditate daily. I love to soak in the bathtub, and I always give myself at least a half an hour longer to meditate and practice guided imagery.

And the thing I do that I recommend for loving and forgiving the negative is practicing mindfulness. Whenever I'm feeling negative, as soon as possible, I sit down and get in touch with those feelings. I treat myself like I would a best friend. No judgment. No criticism. No trying to change how I'm feeling. I tell myself that I accept and love myself just the way I am. I let that part of me know that it is completely safe and loved. I call in spiritual assistance as necessary.

Ken McCaulley once told me a way to deal with negative feelings is to remember that they don't exist in the spiritual dimension. So, welcome them, even cherish them. Whenever you feel depressed for example, tell yourself, "So that's what depression feels like." It's all a matter of perspective.

I found it very interesting that John the Baptist said that it's okay to hate, and have sorrow and pain. Connecting with these through love and acceptance is part of the healing process. John acknowledged that this is difficult, but that even the beautiful rose has thorns. Having faith that life is all unfolding according to Divine Plan can take great trust. And this is all the more difficult when we have had our trust so eroded through childhood and other trauma.

It has been quite a revelation for me to realize that God is truly an intimate part of who we are. Or, more accurately, we are an intimate part of this Divine Source. It is 100% loving, caring, and wise. It only has our best interests in mind and heart. It is easily our best friend. And like John the Baptist, this is the message I want to reemphasize and leave you with: Make time; take time, to connect with the truth of who you are.

Remember – when you know God loves you, you can do anything. This truth will truly set you free. God is not the scary, vengeful, punishing, judgmental Being that many of us were taught. You are indeed loved perfectly, completely. Life serves the purpose of understanding this love more fully. Every one of us, without exception, comes into physical life with a "soul script" and life plan. Life is honestly meant to be joyful, even though the physical plane has its purposeful "negative" aspects. Love is who we are. Love is always the answer. As we live this truth, is it any wonder why love heals?

I've decided to give John the Baptist the last word after all. In reading and rereading what I've written, I admit to some awkwardness writing about spirituality and health. My scientific training and my analytical mind are very evidence driven. I question pretty much everything. How do you prove God?

I also realize that many of you will have come from a traditional religious background. For you, the word God is highly appropriate, and use of other words like Divine Source or any other "New Age" sounding term is quite unacceptable. For others who aren't comfortable with any religious association, the use of the word God creates its own questions and concerns. Of course, whatever God is, it is surely ineffable – beyond any understanding that could be put into words. So, I've asked John the Baptist to define God in a way that I hope has meaning for you:

God is Divine Source. God is not religion. Religion is of man. Divine Source could be best described as the love that comes from, and affects everybody like the rays of sunshine. There is no one that the sun does not touch or have an effect upon. God is True Energy. Energy does not have a beginning or an end such as a vibration. It is eternal. It doesn't matter what man wants to believe or read or practice as his own rituals. Or how he connects with the God Source or Divine Source. That energy is truly within himself. He is God Source.

I can only validate and confirm what you have put in your book: that God is truly Energy. This energy has a Consciousness. It has a connection and a compassion and a love to it. This Energy is not the type of energy that is used on this physical plane to create heat or move something. It has a Consciousness to it that connects to our individual consciousness. It is in its own sense telepathic, where we can have a conversation, and study our intentions. We have an immediate connection to this Consciousness because we are never disconnected from this Source of Consciousness.

I then asked John, "So, we could think of God as Consciousness or Awareness?

Absolutely.

I asked again, "So, another way to refer to God would be Divine Consciousness?"

Absolutely. In fact we really like what you've just said with the term "Divine Consciousness".

Amen. So be it.

Dear reader, this really is the end of the book. However, we'll talk soon in the next book, *John the Baptist Today*.

Index

About the Author

Dean Shrock, Ph.D. attended Cleveland State University, earning a bachelor's degree in psychology. He graduated from the University of Akron in Akron, Ohio with a master's in Community and College Counseling and a doctorate in Counseling Psychology. His doctoral dissertation was titled, *Relaxation, Guided Imagery, and Wellness*.

Dr. Shrock then completed a post-doctoral internship where developed a research proposal for the Cleveland Clinic to test the effectiveness of guided imagery with breast cancer patients. He also interned as a staff psychologist with the Nittany Valley Rehabilitation Hospital in State College, Pa. While there he interned with Dr. Carl Simonton at the Simonton Cancer Center and initiated his research with psychological approaches to cancer care.

Dr. Shrock was then hired by a physician management group to develop and provide psychological services for their cancer centers. Here he developed a wellness program whose primary purpose was to instill a greater "will to live". While bringing more joy and meaning into life surely could affect a patient's quality of life, Dr. Shrock's research published in 1999 found that it extended their length of life. He concluded they lived longer because they felt listened to, cared for and supported. His experience and expertise led to his being invited to co-author the chapter on Mind-Body Medicine in what is regarded as "the definitive source in the field" for healthcare providers, the textbook, *Integrative Oncology*.

Dr. Shrock wrote a book in 2000 about the wellness program he taught and the insights he gained. This book, *Doctor's Orders: Go Fishing*, is not about cancer as much as it is about life. Readers can use the information to get well or stay well.

However, Dr. Shrock was very intrigued by his finding that feeling loved and cared for could extend survival with cancer. This culminated in his 2009 book, *Why Love Heals*. He now resides with his wife, Shelly, in Eagle Point, Oregon, and continues to write and lecture about his "Going Fishing" approach to life, and how to find true joy, peace of mind, great health, and inner love.

Grateful acknowledgement is made for permission to reprint from the following publishers:

Your Soul's Plan: Discovering the Real Meaning of the Life You Planned Before You Were Born by Robert Schwartz, published by Frog Books/North Atlantic Books, copyright © 2009 by Robert Schwartz;

The Divine Matrix by Gregg Braden, published by Hay House, Inc., copyright © 2007 by Gregg Braden;

Ask and It Is Given by Esther and Jerry Hicks, published by Hay House, Inc., copyright © 2004 by Esther and Jerry Hicks;

Everything You Need to Know to Feel Go(o)d by Candace B. Pert, Ph.D., published by Hay House Inc., copyright © 2006 by Candace B. Pert;

Conversations With God: An Uncommon Dialogue, Book 1 by Neale Donald Walsch, copyright © 1995 by Neale Donald Walsch, published by Putnam's Sons, a division of Penguin Group (USA) Inc.;

The Creation of Health by Caroline Myss and C. Norman Shealy, copyright © 1998 by Caroline Myss, Ph.D. and C. Norman Shealy, M.D., Ph.D., published by Three Rivers Press, a division of Random House, Inc.;

Hands of Light by Barbara Ann Brennan, copyright © 1987 by Barbara A. Brennan, published by Bantam Books, a division of Random House, Inc.;

Dr. Dean Ornish's Program For Reversing Heart Disease by Dean Ornish, M.D., copyright © 1996 by Dean Ornish, M.D., published by Ballantine Books, a division of Random House, Inc.;

Getting Well Again by Stephanie Mathews-Simonton, O. Carl Simonton, M.D., and James L. Creighton, copyright © 1978 by O. Carl Simonton and Stephanie Mathews-Simonton, published by Bantam Books, a division of Random House, Inc.;

Quantum Healing by Deepak Chopra, M.D., copyright © 1989 by Deepak Chopra, M.D., published by Bantam Books, a division of Random House, Inc.;

Primary Perception by Cleve Backster, copyright © 2003 by Cleve Backster, published by White Rose Millenium Press;

Soul Medicine by Norman Shealy, M.D., Ph.D. and Dawson Church, Ph.D., copyright © 2006 by C. Norman Shealy and Dawson Church, published by Elite Books;

Other Products by Dean Shrock, Ph.D.

Doctor's Orders: Go Fishing – (soft cover, $16.95)
Describes the program Dr. Shrock taught that affected survival
with cancer. Learn what you can do to improve the quality and
length of your life. Dr. Bernie Siegel said this book is "packed
with wisdom and guidance".

Why Love Heals – (soft cover, $17.95)
Learn why love heals, and how to find true joy, peace of mind,
great health, and inner love. Neale Donald Walsch said, "The
power of human love is made so understandable in [*Why Love
Heals*] that the true wonder is that we don't all immediately fall
in love with each other, and stay in love all the time".

**Guided Imagery for Relaxation and Stress
Management** – (4 guided imagery CD tracks, $14.95)
Learn to create health and happiness in just a few relaxing
minutes. Naturopathic physician, Dr. Tianna Conte, said, "The
sound of his voice and the words of his guided imagery make
this a must listen to CD. Dr. Shrock is a master".

Guided Imagery to Experience Why Love Heals –
(3 guided imagery CD tracks, $14.95)
Experience who you truly are, how the law of attraction really
works, and find your own inner love. Margy Nickelson said, "If
you're wondering what it's all about, here is the answer. *Why
Love Heals* is a must for anyone with questions about
spirituality".

**Dr. Shrock also is available for speaking, workshops
and training events.**

These & Other Products Available At:
www.DeanShrock.com

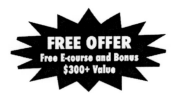

FREE
Special Offer

Lightning Source UK Ltd.
Milton Keynes UK
27 August 2009

143144UK00001B/18/P